Battling Prostate Cancer

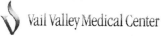

Battling Prostate Cancer
Getting from "Why Me"
to "What Next"

MARVIN A. McMICKLE

Judson Press
Valley Forge

Battling Prostate Cancer: Getting from "Why Me" to "What Next"

Judson Press has made every effort to trace the ownership of all quotes. In the event of a question arising from the use of a quote, we regret any error made and will be pleased to make the necessary correction in future printings and editions of this book.

Bible quotations in this volume (other than those paraphrased by the author) are from *The Holy Bible*, King James Version (KJV); and from the HOLY BIBLE: *New International Version*, copyright © 1973, 1978, 1984. Used by permission of Zondervan Bible Publishers (NIV).

Library of Congress Cataloging-in-Publication Data

McMickle, Marvin Andrew.
Battling prostate cancer : getting from "why me" to "what next" / Marvin A. McMickle.
p. cm.
Includes bibliographical references.
Dealing with the diagnosis — Why me, Lord? — What is prostate cancer? — Which treatment is right for you? — Facing your cancer treatment with faith — You are not alone — Learn from those who have walked by faith — How to reduce your risk of developing prostate cancer — God will never leave us alone.
ISBN 0-8170-1460-8 (alk. paper)
1. Prostate—Cancer—Popular works. 2. Prostate—Cancer—Religious aspects—Christianity. I. Title.
RC280.P7M377 2004
616.99'463—dc22
2004004251

Printed in the U.S.A.
10 09 08 07 06 05 04
10 9 8 7 6 5 4 3 2 1

Dedication

THIS BOOK IS DEDICATED TO CANCER SURVIVORS EVERYWHERE. It is dedicated to the men and women and the boys and girls who are dealing with blood tests, the side effects of surgery, chemotherapy, and radiation, and the hope that their cancer is either in remission, or best of all, has been removed once and for all. It is dedicated to the people who have lost to cancer their hair, organs, control of bodily functions, or dreams and aspirations for the future. If you are alive to read these words, then cancer has not had the final victory in your life. This book is for you.

This book is dedicated to the spouses, families, and loved ones of the victims of cancer. Only they know the full dimensions of the ways in which cancer impacts not only the person whose body carries the disease, but also everyone who is a part of the victim's life in any way. You have stood by and watched while your loved ones have gone through painful, sometimes embarrassing, and often life-altering changes as we have waged our battle with cancer. You know the effects of cancer, whether the cancer has affected the prostate, the breast, the lungs, the uterus, the pancreas, the bones and skeletal structure, the stomach, the skin, or some other part of the body. Your support is invaluable in our recovery process. This book is for you.

This book is dedicated to the members of the medical community in surgery, research, and patient care, who are tirelessly working to bring comfort and cure to the victims of cancer. Your skill as professionals and your deep concern for cancer victims on the human level are a powerful combination, not only in the race for a cure for cancer but, more importantly, in the slow and often painful process of helping cancer victims cope with our condition. Our faith is certainly in God, but many times our bodies are in your hands, and we honor you in those moments when you are the human instruments through which the divine gift of healing flows. This book is for you.

Finally, this book is dedicated to those cancer survivors who have become outspoken advocates for the prevention of this dreaded disease. Someone needs to continually sound the alarm about steps that people can take to safeguard our health and reduce our chances of contracting cancer in the first place. Printed information and television commercials have great affect, but they are no substitute for the testimony of a living, breathing cancer survivor who is willing to stand up before a group and share his or her experiences. This book is intended to do just that on a wider scale, as I urge other men to take steps that can help to prevent them from contracting my kind of cancer. If you are a survivor of any kind of cancer and if you are willing to share your experiences for the benefit of others who can, perhaps, be spared the experiences that we have endured as cancer victims, then I dedicate this book to you as well.

Contents

Foreword

RECEIVING A DIAGNOSIS OF PROSTATE CANCER CAN BE ONE of the most terrifying experiences in a man's life. One very quickly develops a great deal of perspective in terms of what is really important in life. In this book, Marvin McMickle has provided a great service not only by giving men insight into what it is like to experience this diagnosis and its aftermaths, but also by providing valuable information about preventing the development of prostate cancer or at least catching it early when treatment options are best.

Perhaps most importantly, he realizes that our bodies are fearfully and wonderfully made by our Creator and that we are more than physical beings. True healing requires not only physical treatment, but mental and spiritual therapy as well. By combining all three of these aspects in one easily readable volume, he has provided a resource far more valuable than the small amount of money required to purchase it. I hope many men will take advantage of this wealth of information from a man who has turned vulnerability into strength.

—Benjamin S. Carson Sr., M.D.
Director of Pediatric Neurosurgery
Professor of Neurological Surgery
Oncology, Plastic Surgery, and Pediatrics
Johns Hopkins University

Foreword

IN WRITING HIS LATEST ON A MOUNTING LIST OF SIGNIFICANT books, Marvin McMickle speaks to a global audience. To the more than 200,000 men who will be diagnosed with prostate cancer in 2004, Dr. McMickle is teacher, preacher, pastor, and counselor. This pastor, professor, husband, and father has provided an epic treatise on how to be a faithful soldier in battling prostrate cancer.

When Marvin McMickle shared with me in 2003 the challenging news that he had embarked on this battle, we joined in prayer— "fervent, effectual prayer." I then offered to stand in for him as a surrogate preacher for one or more of his Sunday morning worship services. This, to me, was a small act of support and encouragement to Dr. McMickle, his family, and congregation. It was my way of joining the healing team of a friend, colleague, and pastor.

I am honored to write a foreword for this book, which is a profound testimony from one who is a dynamic witness to the power of healing, hope, and health. One cannot read this book without feeling a sense of urgency concerning the whole system of health care in our nation. If Dr. McMickle had been among the more than 40 million uninsured, or the tens of millions of under-insured, his outcome could have been painfully different. The quality of treatment, access to an excellent support structure, and superb post-surgical care would have been missing from the health and treatment equation.

When my good friend Dr. Wyatt Tee Walker of New York returned to active pastoral service after a series of strokes, he wrote a book titled *My Stroke of Grace*. (Dr. Walker is in extensive rehabilitation following additional challenges and retirement plans.) After the late E. Stanley Jones suffered a stroke when he was beyond eighty, he wrote the book *The Divine Yes*. Victor Hugo did some of his best work in exile. Nelson Mandela wrote the first draft of his autobiography while in prison. Wilma Rudolph achieved the Olympic Gold Medal after a battle with polio. Dr. Martin Luther King Jr. did his greatest work and wrote all of his books under constant death threats. The lives of Fannie Lou Hamer and Helen Keller are historic and courageous testimonies of what people can achieve against incalculable odds. Dr. McMickle has taken his battle with cancer and turned it into a blessing and victory of faith, hope, and love in Christ.

This book is a living example of the "wounded healer," a testament to what we can do with our pain and suffering by and through the grace of God, the love of Jesus Christ, the measureless influence of the Holy Spirit, and the presence of a healing community.

Over the past eighteen years Marvin McMickle has preached at Olivet Institutional Baptist Church many times. I have listened to him teach in our annual Spring and Fall Academy, on radio, television, and in many other public venues. He is always uniquely prepared and eloquent. The wisdom and wit he brings to private and public settings have moved many of us. His intellect and spirituality are notably uncommon. Having worked with him on his campaign for U.S. Congress and his subsequent campaign for the U.S. Senate, I know firsthand of his keen debating skills and commitment to thorough research on each subject or issue he addresses.

However, I have noticed a deeper knowledge and a greater power in his preaching since his battle with cancer. There is a dimension of the human spirit that remains unperfected until we have gone through some wilderness of adversity—some desert of agony, some Gethsemane of suffering and sorrow.

One of Dr. Gardner Taylor's seminary classmates and pastoral colleagues often remarked to Dr. Taylor, "Gardner, there is a tear in your preaching." Some of our greatest art, literature, theological, and philosophical depths have come through great pain. Marvin McMickle's book is a product of deep pain.

Gibran poetically and powerfully described life as a "tear and a smile." While this declaration is true, it does not mean that we should go around looking for pain in order to receive spiritual power. But we should embrace the Holy Spirit, who empowers us to convert pain into poetry, haunting fears into hymns of faith, and ashes of agony into garlands of joy. No one should ever go around wishing for cancer, stroke, heart attack, kidney failure, blindness, or paralysis. But we should seek wisdom, grace, and faith to transform our pain into spiritual power, not unto ourselves but to the glory of God.

In years past, preaching in a country church revival, I remember a beautiful saint in her golden years standing in the Amen Corner of that rural church, singing with clarity, power, and melodious beauty: "I'm a soldier!" The congregation responded in unbroken unity, "In the army of the Lord." After several refrains, the dearly beloved saint sang in lowered tones, "I'm a battle-scarred soldier," and the congregation responded, "In the army." After more than four decades, I can still hear and feel that congregation expressing the harmony of shared suffering. In the shared suffering of the community of faith, healing is experienced, and in this experience, medicine and spirituality become abiding friends through God's amazing grace. This is the testimony of Marvin McMickle's book.

Otis Moss Jr.
Senior Pastor
Olivet Institutional Baptist Church
Cleveland, Ohio

Preface

BEING DIAGNOSED WITH PROSTATE CANCER IN THE SPRING of 2003 has changed my life forever. I am now living as a cancer survivor with a commitment to urge other men to be proactive about this aspect of their health care. After undergoing surgery to remove my prostate gland I am now living cancer-free, but I continue to monitor my condition with quarterly blood tests. Most important of all, I live with the knowledge that many men who walked this path ahead of me are now living healthy and happy lives. Many of them, including pastors here in Cleveland and deacons in the church where I serve as pastor, were a great source of support and encouragement for me, especially when I first got the news that I had contracted prostate cancer. Just as those men helped me through my experience, I hope that the information and insights in this book will help you or someone you know and love who is facing a diagnosis of or treatment for prostate cancer.

It has been a little over a year since my diagnosis was confirmed. The day I received that news I had all of the responses you might expect. I wondered if my life was in danger. I wondered if I would be alive even one year later. I asked the question *Why me?* I also began to wrestle with the challenge of moving on to *What next?* As you will discover in this book, these are the steps that you will be encouraged to make: *from "why me" to "what next."*

Prostate cancer is a battle that begins on the day you are diagnosed, and the battle does not end until you are free of the troubling side effects of the treatment option you may choose. In some cases, the side effects last for the rest of your life, and so the battle must be waged every day. The purpose of this book is not merely to present you with the medical facts about prostate cancer—although arming yourself with information about this disease is one important thing you can do both in terms of cancer prevention and cancer treatment. The main purpose of this book is to urge you to call upon your faith in God as you face this life-threatening disease.

There is a familiar song of the black Baptist church that includes this line:

If it had not been for the Lord by my side,
Tell me, where would I be?

I am convinced that the Lord was by my side as I fought my own battle with prostate cancer. It was my faith in God that allowed me to move *from "why me" to "what next."* I hope the experiences and lessons contained in this book will call forth a similar faith from you.

I know better today than I did before I was diagnosed with prostate cancer that I can walk through the valley of the shadow of death and fear no evil because the Lord is with me. This book is meant to be a reminder that God can and will walk with you as well, when you or someone you love engages in a battle with prostate cancer. To paraphrase the words of Paul in 2 Timothy 4, this book is intended to help and encourage you to fight a good fight and keep the faith.

Acknowledgments

THERE ARE MANY PEOPLE I NEED TO ACKNOWLEDGE because without them this book would not have been possible. I begin with my wife, Peggy, who was my primary caregiver at home in the weeks following my surgery. She always wanted to be a nurse in real life, but circumstances prevented that dream from coming true. For six weeks in the summer of 2003, she truly was "Nurse Peggy," and I could not have been in better hands.

I want to thank the members of Antioch Baptist Church of Cleveland, Ohio, who rallied around me when I was diagnosed with prostate cancer and who gave me all the time I needed for my recovery from surgery. I also want to thank the church staff members and the visiting clergy who filled in during my absence from the church and kept everything moving smoothly.

I want to thank Dennis Norris, J. Delano Ellis, David Hunter, Vincent Miller, and Jewel Jones. These men are not only among my pastoral colleagues, but they are also prostate cancer survivors who were immediately and continuously supportive of me through my entire ordeal from detection to diagnosis to treatment and through my ongoing recovery. Their prayers, phone calls, visits, and first-hand testimonies of what it is like to live as a prostate cancer survivor were invaluable and will never be forgotten. I also want to thank those deacons at Antioch Baptist Church who are also prostate cancer survivors for their encouragement and prayerful support.

There is no way to thank Dr. Michael Oefelein enough. He is the urologist who continues to oversee my physical recovery. His good counsel prior to the surgery, his skill in performing the radical prostatectomy, and his follow-up care in the months following my surgery have helped to bring me to where I am today. I also want to thank him for working with me on some medical and technical aspects of this book. His ability as a teacher is as greatly valued as his ability as a surgeon and a patient-care physician.

As always I am indebted to Randy Frame and the people at Judson Press for believing in and supporting this project. Their help in bringing focus to the discussion of prostate cancer in particular, and their assistance in guaranteeing the accuracy of the medical and technical topics discussed in this book have helped to make this a much more useful and reliable resource for persons who are living with or concerned about prostate cancer. This is my fifth project with Judson Press, and with each new book my appreciation increases for the ministry they are performing for the church universal through the National Ministries work of American Baptist Churches USA.

Finally, I want to thank Dr. Ben Carson, himself a prostate cancer survivor, for his willingness to write a foreword for this book. His willingness to speak openly about his experience with prostate cancer was a source of encouragement for me, and his willingness to contribute to this book is an honor for which I will never be able fully to express gratitude. I also want to thank my dear friend and colleague, Rev. Dr. Otis Moss Jr., for his contribution to this book. He is my pastoral colleague on most days and my pastor when I really need someone to talk with about what is happening in my life and ministry. I give thanks to God that our two churches are so close, not only in physical proximity but also in ministry and collaboration.

1

Dealing with the Diagnosis

*We have this treasure in jars of clay to show
that this all-surpassing power is from God and not from us.
We are hard pressed on every side, but not crushed; perplexed,
but not in despair; persecuted, but not abandoned;
struck down, but not destroyed.*
—2 Corinthians 4:7-9, NIV

MY FAMILY HAS A FIRE-RESISTANT LOCKBOX IN WHICH WE keep our birth certificates, insurance policies, passports, and other important documents. Other people, wanting still more protection against fire and loss, rent a safe-deposit box at a bank. Everyone understands that if you want to preserve something, you have to put it away where it will be safe. It's shocking to realize, then, that God does not use the same principle when it comes to the most precious and irreplaceable possessions we will ever have: our life and health.

The apostle Paul said as much when he compared human bodies to the jars of his day that were made with baked clay or mud. God gives us the gift of life and then requires us to house that valuable gift in a fragile container. We do not face each new day of our lives insulated from danger by living inside a box of reinforced steel. Instead, we live out our days within a body that is as easily damaged as a jar of clay.

You and I are not as strong as we think we are. Nor are we as invincible as we wish we were. No matter how hard we work

1

to protect our health, and no matter how unprepared we are to discover that something has gone wrong with our bodies, there are moments in life when we are reminded that our life and health are housed inside a vessel that is prone to pain, sickness, and even death.

I was reminded that my life and health are housed within a jar of clay in February of 2003 when the possibility of prostate cancer was first detected.

The Battle Begins

At the end of my annual physical examination, it seemed I was in good health. The physician had done a digital rectal exam of my prostate gland, and nothing seemed abnormal to the touch. However, several days later, when the results of the blood work were returned to him, he called me on the phone with a level of concern in his voice that I had never heard from him before. He told me that my PSA (prostate-specific antigen) level was elevated with a score of 5.2. He indicated that whenever that number rises above 4.0 he becomes concerned about prostate cancer.

Earlier in 2003 was the first time I had ever spent even one night in a hospital—but now the specter of prolonged hospitalization loomed before me. I had never missed a single day of work as a result of a serious illness. I had always been the picture of health. I was not engaged in any behaviors typically associated with high-risk living—I did not smoke cigarettes or consume large amounts of liquor, for instance. I led an active lifestyle and seemed to have an unlimited level of energy. I went for annual physical exams only as a precaution and never had any severe pains or other physical problems that might indicate that I was contracting a serious illness. I left my doctor's office without a worry in the world about my physical health. I now understand that, prior to my diagnosis, I fit into a category of people who take their good health for granted.

In his book *Not Fade Away: A Short Life Well Lived*, Peter Barton, who was the founder and CEO of the cable TV company Liberty Media, describes his losing battle with stomach cancer. He died from that disease at the age of fifty-two. In that memoir about his living and dying, he says about himself, "I come to realize that up until now I've been guilty of the arrogance of health."[1] That is exactly where I was when I walked out of my primary physician's office after my annual physical. I was not simply in good health; I was guilty of the arrogance of health.

I had never before even considered the possibility of my becoming seriously ill. I was the pastor who went to visit the sick at home or in the hospital. I was the person whose stamina, energy, and active lifestyle were the envy of other people. I took no prescription drugs and had no problem with blood pressure, diabetes, glaucoma, heart disease, or any other life-threatening condition. More importantly, I felt great—no fatigue, no depression, no chronic pain. And having been that way for all of my fifty-four years, I was guilty of the arrogance of health.

Then in one shocking day, following a telephone conversation with my primary physician, I was forced to consider a possibility that had never before entered my mind. I needed further tests to determine if I had contracted cancer. The arrogance of health was shattered and I was coming face-to-face with the fact that I was living inside a jar of clay.

I was referred to a urologist, who began by once again administering the digital rectal exam. He indicated that he thought he felt something out of the ordinary, something that a doctor not specializing in urology might not have detected. After that, he administered an exam that caused a few drops of urine to come out of the tip of the penis onto a plastic strip, which he then examined under a microscope.

3

Given the results of that exam, he decided to begin by treating my condition as prostatitis—an inflammation within the prostate gland that can be resolved through antibiotics. When the number did not drop below 4.0 after one month on the antibiotic, the urologist recommended—and I agreed to—a biopsy of the prostate. Six samples were taken, and when the pathology report was returned, we learned that one of those six samples was cancerous. The urologist now confirmed the red flag of concern that was initially waved by my primary physician back in January: I had developed prostate cancer.

A Word That Hurts Your Ears

I cannot explain the fear and anxiety that suddenly swept over me as I tried to cope with the diagnosis that had just been pronounced. Up to that point in my life, I had suffered with allergies, the common cold, tonsillitis, occasional bouts with the flu, acid reflux, and a painful but easily treatable condition known as paracarditis that was resolved through the use of anti-inflammatory aspirin. Now I was facing something entirely different, something potentially deadly. I had prostate cancer. There was no pill that could fix this problem, and there was no period of time that I had to endure until the sickness would run its course and then leave my body like some bacterial infection.

I do not think that anybody is fully prepared to be told that they have cancer, and I was certainly no exception. There is something about the word cancer and about being diagnosed with cancer that results in almost immediate anxieties about debilitating sickness and unavoidable death. As my son Aaron said when I shared with him the news of my diagnosis, "The word cancer kind of hurts your ears."

The word cancer certainly does "hurt your ears" the first time it is connected to your life and your body. I never dreamed that I would be diagnosed with any kind of cancer. When we hear about most other illnesses, those involving the heart, the arteries, or the limbs and joints, for example, we think about medical techniques that can restore us to health or that can at least allow us to live for many years with the condition. For most people who hear the diagnosis about cancer, though, their thoughts almost immediately turn morbid.

In his book *Now That I Have Cancer—I Am Whole,* John Robert McFarland speaks the sentiments that swept over me and that I suspect sweep over all people when they are first diagnosed with cancer of any kind.

> Cancer makes us think about death, doesn't it? Even if we have every confidence that we shall recover, be cured, be saved from this particular hit man sent by the cancer Mafia, we are reminded that some day we shall die. For many of us, cancer will be the cause of death. Most of us, still, the first time we hear that word applied to us, immediately think of death.[2]

Here again, I was no exception. After receiving the diagnosis of prostate cancer over the phone, I sat in my chair and wondered how much time I had left to live.

The urologist, on the other hand, was anxious to discuss the treatment options that were available to me based upon the stage at which my prostate cancer had been discovered. He was immediately encouraging and wanted to reassure me that my condition was treatable and that I should expect to recover if I moved quickly to take the appropriate action.

I was not yet ready to talk about any next steps or to consider any long-term results of cancer treatment. There was only one thing on my mind, and it would be many days before I could move beyond that one hard, cold reality: I had prostate cancer! I had a date book crowded with appointments and speaking engagements, but now they would have to be put on hold. I had prostate cancer.

I had several writing assignments that I had to complete by their fast-approaching deadlines, but I was suddenly unsure if I would ever complete those projects. I had prostate cancer.

What was going to be the outcome of this unexpected detour into a battle with prostate cancer? All I could do for a few days was sit and wonder, *Am I going to die?* I could not bring myself to stop worrying about my condition. I would sit at my desk and stare at a blank computer screen. I would sit outside on the deck and stare endlessly into space. I knew what Jesus said in Matthew 6:25-34 about the futility of worrying. I knew that by worrying I could not alter my condition one bit. That passage ends with Jesus saying, "Do not worry about tomorrow, for tomorrow will worry about itself. Each day has enough trouble of its own" (verse 34, NIV). Nevertheless, that is exactly where I was on the day I received my diagnosis—that day's troubles seemed more than I could bear.

A Second Opinion

The first thing I did was to get a second opinion from another urologist, hoping against hope that he might review my test results and conclude that the initial diagnosis was wrong and that I did not have cancer. I sought the advice of a urologist whom I had known for several years. I had been well acquainted with his family, who resided in Montclair, New Jersey, during the time when I served as the pastor of a congregation in that city. I had also presided at the wedding ceremony for this young man and his wife. I knew that he would give me an honest opinion and that I could have a frank discussion with him about this matter.

Unfortunately, my friend was not a part of the medical group to which my primary physician belonged, and he also worked at a hospital where my doctor was not on staff. I certainly wanted my own physician to be a part of my medical team as I went through this process, so I decided to remain with the excellent urologist who was not only working in the same hospital as my own primary doctor but who was also on the teaching staff of the local medical school. He was the doctor who had performed all the initial tests and exams, and I had every confidence in his abilities. However, we were talking about my body being infected with cancer, and before I could do anything else, I still had to get a second opinion.

The second opinion confirmed everything that had already been told to me. There was cancer in the tissue taken during the biopsy, and it was aggressive enough to require immediate attention. Both urologists agreed that, given my age and general health, a complete removal of the prostate gland (a procedure called a *radical prostatectomy*) was the best course of action. They also agreed that, in order to minimize the side effects of such a procedure, I should have the nerve-sparing procedure called the *retropubic approach*, which makes the incision into the lower abdomen and looks down directly onto the prostate gland. This is different from the procedure known as the *perineal approach*, which works up through the rectum, with not quite as clear a view of the prostate gland and with an increased risk of some significant permanent side effects, including incontinence and impotence.

Facing the Facts

Long before a cancer patient begins dealing with the treatment regimen, he must come to grips with the fact that he has been diagnosed with cancer. It is a breathtaking and soul-shaking experience. I was encouraged by the fact that my condition was caught in the early stages of cancer before it had spread outside of the prostate. I was encouraged by the fact that many men in my church family and in my other circles of association had already been through that procedure, and their continued good health comforted my troubled spirit. But having said all of that, my first challenge was to come to grips with the fact that this was happening to me.

I had tried to avoid facing up to the possibility that I had cancer. First I tried living in denial, pretending that the news I had just received did not really apply to me. Then I assured myself that the findings were incorrect and that upon a second review of the PSA test and the tissue taken in the second biopsy I would be given a clean bill of health. Finally I turned my prayer life into an urgent appeal to God on a single subject. "Lord, whatever it is that I have, take it away." However, as time went by and the pathology tests were confirmed, one thing became undeniably clear: I did have prostate cancer. God had not taken it away, and this was a battle that I was going to have to face up to and then fight.

How people face up to the fact that they have been diagnosed with cancer greatly influences how they will cope with the treatment options, the side effects of those treatments, and their prospects for recovery and long-term good health. For some people, the discovery that they have cancer of any kind can be enough to send them into hysteria, depression, and a downward spiral of self-pity. For others, that same news can eventually force them to fall back on their faith in God and upon the promises of 2 Corinthians 4:8-9: "We are hard pressed on every side, but not crushed; perplexed, but not in despair; persecuted, but not abandoned; struck down, but not destroyed."

While the first few days after the diagnosis hit me like a ton of bricks, I knew that for several reasons I would have to pull myself together and find a way to face up to the fact that I had cancer. I laid claim to my faith in God and specifically to the promise in 2 Corinthians 4:7-9. I came to believe that while cancer had indeed knocked me down, it would not destroy me. I was clearly perplexed by what was happening to me, but I began to realize that I did not have to be in despair. There is absolutely no doubt in my mind that it was my faith in God's power both to sustain me through my battle with prostate cancer and to eventually heal me from that life-threatening disease that gave me the strength to face up to my cancer diagnosis.

Principles of Pastoral Care

For most of my thirty years of pastoral ministry, I have been informed by what have historically been known as the four steps or stages of pastoral care, which are *healing, guiding, sustaining,* and *reconciling*.[3] There are times in a pastor's life when the object of ministry is to assist people in taking the steps that can result either in their physical healing or in their being reconciled to one another or to an event or circumstance in their lives. Sometimes that reconciliation involves helping people come to an acceptance of some difficulty or trauma they are going to have to endure. Healing and reconciliation are always the long-term goals, but sometimes neither of them is possible, or they are at least not possible at any point in the foreseeable future.

It is when what we want to have happen (healing or reconciliation) is not possible that we need to be guided and sustained until our long-range goals can be achieved or until we can finally face up to a future that is not going to be altered. And it is precisely at times like this that our faith can serve us most effectively. Our faith in God can guide and sustain us until we are healed or until we can be reconciled to the fact that the physical healing we desire is not possible without going through the battle for health that lies before us.

Like anyone else, I would have preferred that God not bring me into a battle with a life-threatening disease. Having said that, I am thankful for the deep reservoir of faith that was already in place in my life, because it was my faith that guided and sustained me during my battle with prostate cancer. I applied to my own life the spiritual principles I had employed as a pastor when I was trying to support persons who were passing through a traumatic period in their lives. Now I was the one passing through a traumatic period, and so I began to draw on that rich and precious resource of faith that was alive and well in my soul. Suddenly I found new meaning in the words "Yea, though I walk through the valley of the shadow of death, I will fear no evil: for thou art with me; thy rod and thy staff they comfort me" (Psalm 23:4, KJV).

My battle with prostate cancer was about to begin, and I had no intention of facing that enemy alone. Neither should you. "The LORD of hosts is with us; the God of Jacob is our refuge" (Psalm 46:7, KJV).

NOTES

1. Laurence Shames and Peter Barton, *Not Fade Away: A Short Life Well Lived* (New York: Rodale, 2003), p. 51.
2. John Robert McFarland, *Now That I Have Cancer—I Am Whole: Meditations for Cancer Patients and Those Who Love Them* (Kansas City, MO: Andrews & McMeel, 1993), p. 81.
3. William A. Clebsch and Charles R. Jaekle, *Pastoral Care in Historical Perspective* (Englewood Cliffs, NJ: Prentice-Hall, 1964), pp. 32–64.

2

Asking, "Why Me, Lord?"

"My grace is sufficient for you,
for my power is made perfect in weakness."
—2 Corinthians 12:9, NIV

I CONFESS THAT INITIALLY I ARGUED WITH GOD ABOUT THE intrusion of prostate cancer into my life, and I tried to point out to God all the reasons why it seemed unfair that I should be faced with this condition. I reminded God that I was the pastor of a congregation that required my time and attention (as if pastors are not supposed to get sick). I reminded God that I tithed on my income (as if my stewardship was supposed to exempt me from the pains and problems of daily life). I even reminded God that my schedule was full of things that I needed and wanted to do, many of them directly touching upon the work of God's kingdom. I didn't have time for cancer, or as the old spiritual put it so well, "I ain't got time to die." My first reaction to the diagnosis of prostate cancer was an angry rebuke directed at God: "Why me?"

That is likely where most people begin when they are diagnosed with any form of cancer. "Why me?" Cancer patients begin by wondering what they may have done, or what they may have failed to do, that has resulted in their ending up with this disease. And with some forms of cancer, there may in fact be some connection between a person's behaviors and the fact that

11

later he or she contracts cancer—one thinks of cigarette smoking and lung cancer. But of course, not all people who smoke cigarettes contract lung cancer, and not everyone who dies from lung cancer was a smoker. Contracting cancer seems to be somewhat capricious, random, and without logic or pattern.

I could not, at the time of my diagnosis, think of anything I had done in the way of diet, behavior, or exposure to any toxic materials that could help explain why I had contracted prostate cancer. The news that I had cancer came to me like a bolt out of the blue. The only question I could think to ask when I was diagnosed with cancer was "Why me?"

At Risk

What I have learned from my reading and from discussions with physicians and other prostate cancer victims is that part of the answer to "Why me?" is that I was in fact at risk for developing this disease. I now know, for instance, that "African American men have the highest risk of developing prostate cancer of any ethnic group in the world."[1] I am African American. I know that a high-fat diet places a man at greater risk for developing prostate cancer.[2] This makes me wonder about every order of a double cheeseburger, with super-sized French fries and a twenty-ounce soft drink, I have consumed over my lifetime. I know that men over fifty enter a stage in life when they are increasingly at risk of developing this disease.[3] I was diagnosed at the age of fifty-four. I also know that prostate cancer can run on both your father's and your mother's side of the family, and if "your father or your brother has had prostate cancer, your risk of developing the disease is twofold greater."[4] My father did die of cancer, but he never told us (and I never thought to ask him) what type of cancer he had developed.

12

For many reasons, then, I was at high risk for prostate cancer. But all of this is a matter of retrospect. If I knew ten to fifteen years ago what I know now about prostate cancer, I might have been able to reduce my chances of getting this disease. But I was not aware of these things during the time in my life when knowing them could have made a big difference. All I knew at the time of my diagnosis was that I had developed prostate cancer. And all I wanted to know was "Why me?"

Why Me?

Let me suggest that while people who are diagnosed with cancer may start with "Why me?" and with other words of self-pity, that is not where they should remain for long. This is especially true if they are Christians and believe, in the words of Romans 8:28, that "all things work together for good to them that love God, to them who are called according to [God's] purpose" (KJV). The words "Why me?" are a cry of shock, desperation, self-pity, and fear. More importantly, the words "Why me?" focus on the present moment. They cause us to consider only what we have just been told, and they effectively prevent us from considering what good medicine and a gracious God can accomplish, despite our being diagnosed with a potentially deadly disease.

In truth, there is no more selfish question to direct toward God than the words "Why me?" In a world where everybody faces some kind of hardship or suffering at some point in their lives, the words "Why me?" imply that we should somehow be exempt from that hard reality. Why should other people be confronted with sickness and death while I am forever spared those realities? Why should other families be plagued with pain and problems while my family is left unscathed? Why should the people to whom I minister have to adjust their lives to the intrusion of an unexpected and deadly diagnosis while I sail along untouched and untroubled?

Rabbi Harold Kushner has written a book entitled *When Bad Things Happen to Good People.*[5] What he approaches as a legitimate question Jesus addresses as an absolute fact. In John 16:33 Jesus speaks these words to his disciples: "In this world you will have trouble" (NIV). Sickness, suffering, pain, and problems are not the exception to the rule of life; they *are* the rule of life. "In this world you will have trouble," and neither fame nor fortune nor even deep faith in God can buy any one of us an exemption from this fact.

You may not be diagnosed with prostate cancer or any other form of cancer or physical sickness. But that does not mean that you will not have to face trouble in some other form. The words spoken by Jesus in John 16:33 seem to have been true for all the major characters of the Bible. If the reality of trouble was true for them, why should it be any different for us? Abraham and Sarah had to endure various trials; why not us? Moses and the people he led from slavery to freedom had to endure hard trials; why not us? King Hezekiah was faced with the prospect of a sickness that would end his life; why not us? The family of Ruth was acquainted with grief. David's family knew hardships from one generation to the next. "In this world you will have trouble."

"Why me?" is as selfish a question as can be raised by a Christian. According to John 11:35, Jesus wept at the grave of his friend Lazarus; why should we expect to be spared from tears and grief and sorrow? Paul struggled with a thorn in his flesh, which we presume to have been some physical ailment. On three occasions he asked God to remove it, but the only answer he received was "My grace is sufficient for you" (2 Corinthians 12:9, NIV). John was imprisoned on the isle of Patmos, and his brother James was killed with a sword by order of Herod. If God did not exempt them from the troubles of life, why would we imagine that we should be exempted?

Why *Not* Me?

The question of "Why me?" must initially be replaced by the observation "Why *not* me?" If David had to shed tears over the death of his son Absalom, why not me as I confront whatever events might bring tears to my eyes? If Job or Habakkuk had to wonder aloud where God was while their lives seemed to be overwhelmed with sickness and sorrow, why not me as I struggle to cope with sickness and the sorrow that occasionally sweeps over my soul? If blind Bartimaeus had to feel his way into the presence of Jesus, and if the woman with an issue of blood that had lasted for twelve years turned to Jesus with a sense of anxiety and desperation, why not me as I struggle to cope with the news that I have joined the ranks of cancer patients?

The first step in the battle with prostate cancer, or with any other cancer or life-threatening condition, is to move away from self-pity and the quest for sympathy, recognizing that our condition is not unique. The moment that I shared with my congregation that I had been diagnosed with prostate cancer, I was overwhelmed by the number of men both in the church and within the wider community who shared with me the fact that they, too, had battled the disease. What was happening to me has happened to many others. In fact, about 220,900 men are diagnosed with prostate cancer, and about 28,900 men die from this disease every year.[6]

When you are diagnosed with prostate cancer, the question should not be "Why me?" The better observation is "Why *not* me?" Bad things really do happen to good people, and from time to time they will happen to you and me. The first real challenge involves how we respond to the diagnosis when it comes. The question "Why me?" tends to freeze you in a moment in time and all you can do is sit there and consider your condition. The question "Why not me?" links you to the tens of thousands of other men who have shared or do share that same condition, and in so doing it also serves to remind you that your condition is not unusual, untreatable, or incurable. The moment I shifted from self-pity to recognition of the facts and the awareness that I was not alone, I was ready and able to face head-on my battle with prostate cancer.

What Next?

The third and final question that I had to answer was how I was going to wage my battle against prostate cancer. There was one more step I knew I had to take after my cancer diagnosis was confirmed, and that step involved the question "What next?" The first step was the time of self-pity and regret known as "Why me?" The second step was the realization that bad things do happen to good people, and God had not failed me just because I had developed prostate cancer. Therefore, I was free to look myself in the mirror and say, "Why *not* me?" However, in the months between the diagnosis and the actual surgery, the final hurdle I had to cross involved what I was going to do and how I was going to behave during that period of time.

Once you have had a biopsy of the prostate gland, you cannot have the prostate removed for at least two months. You have to give that area of your body time to heal from the trauma and bleeding that are results of having had those six to eight tissue specimens removed. This is true, I discovered, even though you will eventually have the prostate gland removed. My prostate cancer was confirmed in mid-May of 2003, but my surgery date was set for July 31, 2003. I had all of that time in between to try and live a somewhat normal life while knowing that I was living with a cancer that was serious enough to require surgical treatment.

That was the hardest part of the process for me, because during those two months, all I could do was wait for the time to pass and wonder what would be the outcome. Two months is a long time to think, and it is even longer when you are thinking about whether you are going to be alive much longer. I knew that how I spent those two months between the biopsy and the surgery would be crucial in many ways, and so I had to make a decision about what I would do with that time. That is what I mean by the question of "What next?"

Practicing What I Preach

I have been in the pastoral ministry since 1973 and have served as a senior pastor since 1976. In all of those years, I have comforted and consoled dozens of men who had to cope with the news that they had contracted prostate cancer. If you were to add breast cancer, colon cancer, lung cancer, brain cancer, cervical cancer, stomach cancer, testicular cancer, skin cancer, and any of the other forms of cancer that people can develop, I have comforted hundreds of people who were given the diagnosis of cancer. I have listened to their concerns. I have offered my support and encouragement. I have prayed with them as they thought about what their next course of action would be. However, in those instances I was never the person who was forced to deal with the diagnosis of cancer. I was an interested and concerned observer, but I was not the person left wondering how rapidly the cancer might be spreading through my body.

All of that changed when I received my diagnosis. Cancer had not invaded the body of one of my church members or that of one of my friends or family; this time it had happened to me.

I knew that I had to turn this experience of cancer into an opportunity for ministry. I knew that every member of my congregation would be looking at me to see how I was going to handle this experience. I knew that people who lived all over Greater Cleveland would be watching to see if I would be able to practice in my own life what I had been preaching to them for eighteen years: "The Lord will make a way somehow."

A special burden falls upon persons who are in church leadership positions and who are suddenly brought face-to-face with sickness or suffering or sadness. People want to see if we will crumble under the pressure of that pain, in large part because they have repeatedly heard us challenge them not to do so when we were walking with them through a similar experience. In a sense, my future effectiveness in ministry was as much on the line as was my physical health. That is why there was so much urgency attached to the question of "What next?"

If I were to panic, become distraught, appear to be in desperation, and show no early evidence of trust in God, I would have been hard pressed to challenge anybody else to show faith at some point in the future when troubles came their way. I knew almost at once that it was time for me to practice in my own life what I had been preaching to others all these years. It was for all of these reasons that I earnestly asked God to give me the strength and confidence to demonstrate to others a spiritual discipline that I call being "sick and saved."

Certainly this is one of the ways by which we Christians can and should distinguish ourselves from the world around us. All people are likely to get sick at some point in our lives; there is no safeguard against that. The difference should be noticeable when it comes to the manner in which we bear up under our sickness. To be sick is a description of our physical condition. To be sick and saved is a description of our spiritual condition. To be sick is to describe what is happening inside our body, but to be sick and saved is to describe how our faith will enable us to confront and even to combat our sickness.

Here was a chance for me to live out a sermon that would have far more power than any sermon I could deliver with mere words. I was sick and saved; therefore, I would not be engulfed in self-pity. I was sick and saved; therefore, I would speak about and exhibit my faith in God to bring me through this experience. I was sick and saved; therefore, I would face the future with hope and confidence. I was not merely sick, because that description gave too much power to my prostate cancer diagnosis. I was sick *and* saved, and that allowed me the chance to demonstrate in my own life things I had only heard others speak about in prayer meetings. The Lord will make a way somehow.

During my time of sickness, I gave a great deal of thought to Paul's encounter with Christ as recorded in 2 Corinthians 12:7-10. Paul was asking Christ to remove his "thorn in the flesh." Nobody knows exactly what that thorn was, but three times Paul asked that it be removed. That is how I first began dealing with my own sickness—I asked God to remove it. After the PSA test, but before the biopsy, I asked God to remove the sickness from me, but God didn't do that. After I had the biopsy, but before the results came back, I asked God to remove the sickness, but God didn't do that. After the biopsy results came back, but before I went for a second opinion, I asked God to remove the sickness, but again God didn't do that.

God's answer to my repeated prayers was no. However, just because God does not choose to keep us from serious illness does not mean that God has failed us. Sometimes, as with the decision by Jesus not to heal Lazarus but to raise him from the dead instead (John 11:4), God wants to get glory out of certain situations. That glory is not possible if God always keeps us from something, but it can occur when God decides to bring us through something. Here is where the power to be sick and saved resides. "My grace is sufficient for you, for my power is made perfect in weakness."

Sharing the News

The principle of being sick and saved helped me to make another major decision that confronted me in the weeks and months that followed my diagnosis. I struggled with the question of whether I should I keep this news to myself or share it with others outside my immediate family. I could have had the operation and gone through the recommended six-week recovery period during the summer months when my absence could have been explained away as a prolonged vacation. No one would have wondered or complained about that.

In the end, I decided against secrecy and chose instead to use this experience as an opportunity for congregational pastoral care. I preached a series of sermons in the month of July leading up to my surgery on July 31, 2003. My objectives in each of those sermons were to talk openly about my prostate cancer diagnosis, to urge other men in the church to be screened for prostate cancer, and to invite the church to pray for me as I had so often prayed for them in the face of sickness. I also wanted to challenge them to face similar experiences in their lives with the openness and confidence that I was trying to demonstrate before them.

How could I demonstrate the model of being sick and saved if I chose to handle the experience secretly? I know many other men who did decide to keep their battle with prostate cancer a secret, at least until after their recovery from whatever treatment they had selected. That was not my choice, however, because by being open about my diagnosis and the surgery that I was facing, I was able to turn a personal sickness into a marvelous ministry opportunity with the members of my congregation.

Watchman, What of the Night?

The next step in my journey from "Why me?" to "What next?" involved deciding whether it would be helpful to talk about my battle against prostate cancer with people beyond the Antioch Baptist Church family. Prostate cancer is rampant in the African American community nationwide. Men like Harry Belafonte, Minister Louis Farrakhan, Dr. Ben Carson, and many other prostate cancer survivors had made the decision to speak publicly about their battle in the hope that they could increase awareness about the dangers of prostate cancer and about the importance of being screened for this life-threatening disease. In fact, I have a photograph of me standing with Harry Belafonte on the day he spoke about his battle with this disease from the Antioch pulpit to a packed house of men from our congregation and from the Greater Cleveland community. He spoke widely about his experience; was this something I should be willing to do as well?

In Isaiah 21:11 we find the phrase "Watchman, what of the night?" (KJV). In that passage and in Ezekiel 3 and Ezekiel 33, the idea of the watchman is employed. The job of the watchman was to remain vigilant and attentive to any dangers that might be approaching the city and to sound the alarm if any such danger came into sight. A staggering number of men are contracting prostate cancer in the United States. I remind you again: the American Cancer Society confirms that about 220,900 new cases of the disease are reported every year and about 28,900 men die annually from prostate cancer. Yet there is still not nearly enough public discussion about the dangers posed by this disease or its impact upon our families and our society. The fact that I had been diagnosed with prostate cancer forced me to ask myself whether God was putting me in a "Watchman, what of the night?" position.

I made up my mind that if God were to open up an opportunity for me to talk about my own experience to an even wider audience, I would do so. Much to my surprise, one week before my surgery was scheduled, a reporter from the local black community newspaper, *The Call and Post*, was sitting in my office to interview me about my recently released book on premarital counseling, entitled *Before We Say I Do.*[7] At the end of the interview, he casually asked me about my health since he had heard that I had been hospitalized earlier that year for chest pains. (It ended up being a case of pneumonia coupled with a buildup of fluid around my heart and a condition known as *paracarditis.*) Here was the opportunity that God was providing, if only I had the courage and willingness to use it.

For the next hour the reporter and I embarked upon what amounted to a second interview. He then came to the church on July 27, 2003, to hear the last of the sermons that I was to preach before I went into the hospital for the surgery. He ran a two-page story in the newspaper while I was at home recovering from my surgery.[8] I am still running into men who say they rushed out and got screened for prostate cancer after reading that story in the newspaper. Women gave that story to their husbands and urged them to get screened for this disease.

I thank God for opening that window of opportunity to share my message about prostate cancer with a much wider audience than I ever could have reached on my own. When I realize that God has used my battle with prostate cancer to alert other men and their families to the dangers of prostate cancer, and also to the steps that can be taken to reduce their risk of developing this disease, I am all the more grateful that I made the move from "Why Me?" to "Why *not* me?" to "What next?" I believe, more than ever, that God has a purpose for the things God allows to happen in our lives, if we can just look beyond self-pity and see our experiences, even our experiences with cancer, as ministry opportunities. I have a new appreciation for Romans 8:28, which says, "We know that all things work together for good to them that love God, to them who are called according to his purpose" (KJV).

By God's Grace

As a result of my battle with prostate cancer, I have learned that the words of Jesus in John 16:33 apply to every one of us, Christians and non-Christians alike: "In this world you will have trouble." What remains to be seen is whether we can take comfort in the words of Jesus that come next in that passage: "But take heart! I have overcome the world" (NIV). This is possible for those who put their faith in God as revealed through Jesus Christ. Tribulations will surely come, sometimes in the form of prostate cancer or other life-threatening diseases. When they do, we may initially be stunned and frightened by the prospects that confront us. "Why me?" and "Am I going to die?" are common responses when we first receive the news that we have cancer. Even the strongest and most devout Christian may initially be overwhelmed by this diagnosis. What we will need to do at some point is begin to let our faith in God go to work for us.

We will need to remind ourselves of the words of Paul in 2 Corinthians 12:9 that says, "My grace is sufficient for you, for my power is made perfect in weakness" (NIV). Prostate cancer can leave us feeling weak and overwhelmed, but if we are sick *and* saved, then our faith in God will surely equip us for the battle with prostate cancer that lies ahead.

Notes

1. Patrick Walsh and Janet Farrar Worthington, *Dr. Patrick Walsh's Guide to Surviving Prostate Cancer* (New York: Warner, 2001), p. 40.
2. Sheldon Marks, *Prostate and Cancer: A Family Guide to Diagnosis, Treatment, and Survival* (Cambridge, MA: Fisher, 1999), pp. 25–27.
3. Walsh and Worthington, *Dr. Patrick Walsh's Guide,* p. 40.
4. Ibid., pp. 40–41.
5. Harold S. Kushner, *When Bad Things Happen to Good People* (New York: Avon, 1981).
6. American Cancer Society, *Cancer Facts and Figures, 2003,* pp. 10, 16.
7. Marvin A. McMickle, *Before We Say I Do: Seven Steps to a Healthy Marriage* (Valley Forge, PA: Judson, 2003).
8. Eric Heard, "Practicing What You Preach, Even When It Is Done from the Valley of the Shadow of Death," *The Call and Post,* magazine supplement, August 7, 2003, pp. 8–9.

3

Understanding Prostate Cancer

My people are destroyed for lack of knowledge.
—Hosea 4:6, KJV

TO START YOUR BATTLE WITH PROSTATE CANCER AS WELL as to make the adjustment from "Why me?" to "What next?" begin by learning as much as you can about this disease. The purpose of this chapter is to help you with that. I am not writing for the consumption of medical professionals; instead, my target audience is the average man who is likely to be diagnosed with prostate cancer and who wants to learn more about the disease from the perspective of someone who has had it.

I want to discuss the issue in terms of three separate topics. The first is a definition of prostate cancer. The second topic is the process by which prostate cancer is detected. The third topic involves the steps necessary to reach an accurate diagnosis of prostate cancer.

Here is a case where knowledge truly is power. The more a person knows about prostate cancer, the more likely it is that he will be able to win the battle against this potentially life-threatening disease. It is important for men to learn as much as possible about prostate cancer as soon as possible and not wait until they begin to feel symptoms associated with the disease. By the time someone feels the symptoms, it may already be too late for him to be cured.

Let me repeat that a man's chances of contracting prostate cancer are influenced by issues of family history, racial ancestry, diet, and lifestyle. The chance of developing prostate cancer increases as a man gets older. It is rarely seen in men under the age of fifty, but the chances of developing the disease are greatly increased among men over fifty. The vast majority of cases (80 percent) occur in men over the age of sixty-five. The question of age is important where prostate cancer is concerned because the patient's age and the stage at which his prostate cancer is detected will influence the kind of treatment his doctor might recommend.

In some cases, prostate cancer treatment can have some embarrassing and frustrating side effects. Among them are incontinence (a loss of urinary control) and impotence (the inability to have or maintain an erection). If the cancer is detected early enough, and if an appropriate treatment plan is followed, these conditions can be reversed. If the cancer is left untreated, the disease can become more life threatening and the side effects of the medical procedures are less likely to be reversed.

The more you know about prostate cancer, and the sooner you act upon what you know, the more likely it is that you can reduce your chances of contracting this disease or that you can detect your disease at an early stage so that treatment can result in a cure. The prophet Hosea was right when he said, "My people are destroyed by a lack of knowledge." He was directing his comments to some of the priests of ancient Israel who were misleading the nation by their words and deeds. Had the people known more, they might have behaved differently. I am appropriating this verse from Hosea 4:6 and applying it to the battle with prostate cancer. I do not want another man to be destroyed by prostate cancer due to a lack of knowledge. This book is written with that hope in mind.

Pay Attention!

Unfortunately, I did not take the time to learn any of the things that will be discussed in this chapter prior to my own diagnosis, and nobody ever took the time to explain to me why I should. I paid little attention to the issue of prostate cancer until my primary physician told me about my elevated PSA score. I had been screened for prostate cancer on several occasions by my own physician as well as by urologists who had come out to the community on several occasions to offer free digital rectal exams. In each of those earlier instances I was told that I had nothing to be concerned about, so I gave the matter no further thought.

In retrospect, I should have been learning about prostate cancer from the time I turned forty years of age. That way I could have been focused for the next decade on the prevention of prostate cancer, rather than dealing with treatment options once the disease had been detected.

As soon as my primary care physician voiced the concern that I might have prostate cancer, I set out to learn as much about this condition as possible. I wanted to be equipped with information before I went to see the urologist who would do all of the specialized tests and make the final determination of whether cancer was present in the prostate gland. I reasoned that if I knew more about this disease and its effects, I would know what to ask and what to expect from that encounter. Sadly, that was all reactive and after the fact of having contracted the disease. Had I known then what I know now about prostate cancer, I might have been able to avoid, or at least greatly delay, this whole episode.

While it is too late for me to personally benefit from this knowledge, I am determined to share this information with as many men and their families as possible. I cannot turn back the clock on my own experience, but, to paraphrase the Christian hymn, if I can help someone else as I pass along, then my battle with prostate cancer will not be in vain.

Sources of Information

My information came from three primary sources, and these sources are likely to be as reliable for other men as they were for me. The sources were fellow prostate cancer sufferers, books on prostate cancer, and informational websites focused on prostate cancer and its defeat.

My first round of discussions was with other men who had already been through a battle with prostate cancer. I wanted a first-hand description of the problem. Only after I had publicly announced my diagnosis did some of the men with whom I spoke reveal that they, too, had been through a battle with prostate cancer. I was amazed to discover how many men in my local church and in my various civic and fraternal circles had been through some form of prostate cancer treatment. I was able to learn from them their experiences with the various methods of treating this disease, and I was able to discuss the way each of them experienced some of the side effects of the treatment they underwent. It was extremely encouraging to me to speak with these prostate cancer survivors (many of whom had been treated for the disease between one and fifteen years earlier) because they were my living reminders that I, too, could survive my battle with prostate cancer.

I was not the only one who had to face this challenge; men all around me had successfully come through what I was now facing. Their survival and their willingness to share their experiences with me kept me encouraged as I faced up to and then began to decide how to respond to the fact that I had developed prostate cancer. This greatly helped me in my transition from "Why me?" to "What next?" I realized I was not the only man to develop this disease. (That helped with the "Why me?" question.) Now I saw all of these men who had been treated for the same condition at various times in the past and were thriving. (That went a long way to helping me get to the "What next?" step in my own battle with prostate cancer.)

After speaking with other men about their experiences with prostate cancer, I read materials that had been produced by the American Cancer Society and the National Cancer Institute dealing with prostate cancer.[1] I also turned to two books by urologists who are leading experts on the treatment of prostate cancer. The first book was *Prostate and Cancer: A Family Guide to Diagnosis, Treatment, and Survival,* by Sheldon Marks.[2] The second book was *Dr. Patrick Walsh's Guide to Surviving Prostate Cancer* by Patrick Walsh and Janet Farrar Worthington.[3]

Finally I turned to several Internet locations for even more information. These included the following:

- American Cancer Society (www.cancer.org)
- American Foundation for Urologic Disease (www.afud.org)
- American Prostate Society (www.ameripros.org)
- National Cancer Institute (www.cancer.gov/newscenter)

Definitions

Before we go any further, it is important to make sure we are understanding some key terms related to prostate cancer. Consider the following definitions.

What is the prostate?

The prostate is a walnut-sized gland within the male reproductive system. This gland is located just below the bladder and in front of the rectum. It is wrapped around a tube called the urethra that carries urine and semen out of the penis. The principal job of the prostate is to provide fluid for sperm.

From birth until adolescence, the prostate is small, but it doubles in size during puberty. Then it can begin growing again at around age forty or forty-five, and it can continue to grow for the rest of a man's life. This growth in the size of the prostate gland is usually the result of cells creating a condition known as benign prostatic hyperplasia, or BPH. This is not a cancerous condition, but it often results in blockage of the normal flow of urine through the prostate and the urethra and it can be quite painful.[4]

According to the National Cancer Institute, many men who experience this condition report the following symptoms:

- a slow or weak urinary stream
- awakening repeatedly at night to urinate
- pain while attempting to urinate
- an inability to pass urine out of the body
- blood in the urine or semen
- pain during ejaculation
- frequent pain or stiffness in the lower back, hips, or upper thighs
- persistent and prolonged pain in the pelvic area
- loss of appetite and weight

While these symptoms can occur in men who are later diagnosed with prostate cancer, they are most often indicators of BPH. They can also be associated with another prostate condition called prostatitis, which is an inflammation of the prostate that can be treated with an antibiotic.[5]

What is prostate cancer?

Cancer is a condition that results when the normal production of cells is disrupted and the body begins to produce more cells than are needed. Those excess cells form into a mass of tissue that can become a tumor. That tumor can continue to enlarge, pressing against vital organs of the body.

A tumor can be either benign or malignant. If it is benign, that means it will not invade nearby tissue or spread to other parts of the body. If it is malignant, however, the cells will continue to grow out of control and will invade other tissue and possibly enter the bloodstream or the lymphatic system.

Most forms of cancer are named for the type of cell or organ in which they begin. Prostate cancer is a malignant growth of cells within the prostate gland. Like all cancers, it probably starts out as a tiny change within just a few cells of the prostate. Over many years, these cells can develop into a cluster that gradually enlarges within the gland. As the cancer cells multiply, the spread of the cancer in the prostate gains momentum, spreading more widely throughout the prostate.

If the cancer is detected and treated while it is limited to the prostate gland, the prospects for a good recovery from the disease are quite high.[6] If not detected and treated in time, on the other hand, the cancer can begin to spread outside the prostate gland, attaching itself to the bladder, the lymph nodes, or the bones of the rib and pelvic areas. Once the cancer has spread outside the prostate and has metastasized or become embedded in the tissue, organs, and bones around the prostate, the prospects for healing are limited. At that point the focus usually shifts to pain management and trying to keep the patient comfortable as he endures the effects of the cancer.[7]

The fact that the prostate gland sits in the midst of so many other vital parts of the body to which it can spread, resulting in an even more life-threatening condition, is the greatest argument for men to seek an early detection of this condition. Prostate cancer can be treated and cured if it is caught early, when the cancer cells are still contained within the prostate itself. Men need to begin screening for prostate cancer once a year when they reach the age of forty-five or fifty. African American men, being twice as likely to contract prostate cancer (for reasons of genetics and possibly a high-fat diet), should begin screening for prostate cancer every year once they turn forty.

How prevalent is prostate cancer?
Prostate cancer is the second most common type of cancer among men, after skin cancer. It is also the second leading cause of cancer death in men, exceeded only by lung cancer. As mentioned previously, about 220,900 new cases of prostate cancer are diagnosed each year in the United States. On average, 28,900 deaths every year in this country are attributed to prostate cancer. Prostate cancer accounts for 33 percent of all male cancers and 10 percent of all male cancer-related deaths.[8]

Who is most at risk for contracting prostate cancer?
This form of cancer can occur in men of all ages, but it occurs more often in men over the age of fifty, and it occurs most often in men over the age of sixty-five. Three out of four newly diagnosed cases of prostate cancer occur in men over the age of sixty-five.

The highest rates of prostate cancer occur in North America and in northwestern Europe. The disease is rare among men in Asia and Central and South America. The highest rates of infection globally are among men of sub-Saharan African descent. According to the American Cancer Society,

African American men are more likely to develop prostate cancer and have poorer survival rates for prostate cancer than white Americans. In part, this is because prostate cancers in African Americans are often found in advanced stages compared with cancers in white Americans. Because of their greater risk of getting this disease and poorer survival rates after the cancer is found, African American men are more than twice as likely to die of prostate cancer than are white men.[9]

Genetics and diet are believed to be significant factors in determining whether a person contracts prostate cancer. Men whose fathers have had prostate cancer are at a higher risk of the disease. The younger the father was when he was detected with the disease, the greater the odds are that the sons will also contract prostate cancer.[10] In addition to genetics, some studies suggest that a high-fat diet increases a man's chances of contracting prostate cancer.

Detection of Prostate Cancer

The American Cancer Society says that the best defense is early detection.[11] The earlier prostate cancer is found, the better the chances will be that it can be treated and that the man involved can live a healthy and productive life.

Two tests are used to detect prostate cancer; they are the *digital rectal exam (DRE)* and a blood test called the *prostate-specific antigen (PSA)* test. It is strongly recommended that men who have taken the digital rectal exam also get the PSA blood test. As I noted, in my case, my physician did not detect anything abnormal during the DRE, but he was alerted to a possible problem by the results of the blood test.

The digital rectal exam (DRE). The digital rectal exam involves a physician reaching a finger through the rectum and physically examining the prostate for any abnormally firm areas or any irregular growths that might indicate the presence of a cancerous tumor within the prostate. Many men resist this procedure because they are self-conscious about or uncomfortable with the idea of someone probing through their rectum in order to reach the prostate. It is not a comfortable procedure to undergo, but it should be an essential part of the annual physical checkup of men upon reaching the age when they could be at risk (between ages forty-five or fifty for most men; for African Americans, especially those with a family history, at age forty).

The prostate-specific antigen blood test (PSA). The PSA blood test is an exam that looks for a certain protein in the blood. A PSA test result between 0 and 3.9 is considered to be within the normal range. A level above 4 raises concern.

If a man's PSA level is found to be high, the first thing he should do is have the test repeated. Several factors can result in an elevated PSA level, including inflammation of the prostate and even the DRE. The PSA exam has frequently been criticized because it yields a false positive reading or a false negative reading in from 10 percent to 20 percent of the men who are tested. However, the rate of deaths related to prostate cancer has gone down steadily since 1996, when the PSA test began to be widely used.[12]

Having the PSA screening done every year offers a clear benefit. PSA levels in healthy men tend to remain relatively stable, rising only gradually from year to year. The presence of cancer cells and the protein they produce in the blood causes the PSA level to rise more dramatically. Men who tend not to get annual physical exams, including the DRE and the PSA exam, place themselves at greater risk for detecting prostate cancer at later and more life-threatening stages. Again, the best defense against late-stage prostate cancer is early detection.

Diagnosis of Prostate Cancer

The two exams that have just been discussed may detect the presence of prostate cancer, but they are not the ultimate way by which cancer is officially diagnosed. When either your DRE or your PSA level raises concern for you and your physician, it is probably time to have a biopsy performed on the prostate gland.

A biopsy is a test in which a needle is inserted through a probe that reaches through the rectum and into the prostate. First the prostate is examined through the use of an ultrasound that allows any infected areas to be detected visually. Then six to eight tissue samples of those areas are taken by the needle and sent off to a pathology lab for analysis. The pathology report finally and officially determines whether cancer is present in the prostate gland.[13]

It should be remembered throughout this process that a high PSA number is a warning sign that cancer *might* be present in your prostate gland, not a determination that it is present. I know of many men who have high PSA numbers but whose biopsies determined that they had no cancer in any of the sampled tissue. For example, one man with a PSA number of 24 has had his prostate biopsied on four different occasions over a ten-year period, and cancer has never been detected. (On the other hand, I had a relatively low PSA number of 5.2, which came down to 4.7 after it was treated with antibiotics for a month. However, cancerous cells were found in one of the samples taken during my biopsy.) So do not panic if your PSA number is elevated; that is not the definitive sign of cancer.

The digital rectal exam alone cannot detect prostate cancer, and that is largely because the physician cannot feel all parts of the gland. You must follow up the DRE with the PSA blood test. The PSA blood test may indicate that something has caused your prostate gland to become enlarged or infected; however, that does not mean that you have cancer. Only a biopsy and microscopic examination of tissue samples can determine with certainty that cancer is or is not present.

The Gleason Score

If it is determined that you do have prostate cancer, it is important that you know how aggressive or malignant your cancer is so that a course of action can be planned to either cure you from cancer or control its spread and the pain that an aggressive cancer can cause. Tissue samples are graded for their aggressiveness through a standardized measurement called the Gleason score. When a sample of your tissue taken in the biopsy is analyzed under a microscope, the pathologist is looking for two things: how the cells look and how the cells are arranged. The cells are graded with a score of from 1 to 5 with these two factors in mind. Those two numbers, when added together, become the Gleason score.

A Gleason score can range from 2 to 10, and the higher that number is, the more aggressive the cancer is. Based upon the Gleason score, the cancer cells are assigned a grade, and that grade indicates how advanced and aggressive the cancer is. The three grades of prostate cancer are called *low-grade cancer, intermediate cancer,* and *high-grade cancer.* Determining the grade of your cancerous tissue is vitally important because it helps you and your physician determine the amount of cancer that is in the prostate gland and what treatment plans should be considered.[14]

Low-grade prostate cancer. Low-grade prostate cancer is the least dangerous form, usually carrying a Gleason score of from 2 to 4. The cells appear to be normal both in their shape and in the way they are arranged inside the tissue. Those cells are considered to be well differentiated. The cancer has not become aggressive, and it is not showing signs of rapid growth. It is likely that more aggressive forms of cancer start at this level, and should that low-grade cancer go undetected or untreated, the cells will continue to grow and enlarge.

Often no treatment beyond medication is recommended for a low-grade cancer. However, you would be wise to remain watchful of this condition, continuing to monitor your PSA score on a regular basis to be sure it is not getting higher. You might also want to have another biopsy done at a time that you and your urologists have agreed upon. Remember that all prostate cancers begin as low grade, but if left undetected or untreated, they continue to grow and expand, first within the prostate itself and then beyond that to the surrounding bone, tissue, and lymph nodes. After early detection, continued monitoring is essential.

Intermediate prostate cancer. A Gleason score of from 5 to 7 is considered a moderate or intermediate case of prostate cancer. This is the grade of prostate cancer that most men have when they get their pathology diagnosis. Cancer cells in this range can behave like a low-grade or like a high-grade cancer. That means they could continue to grow very slowly and not require any immediate attention, or they could expand to a life-threatening size if they remain untreated. Urologists suggest that intermediate-grade prostate cancer be treated as if the potential for aggressive growth is there.[15]

High-grade prostate cancer. High-grade prostate cancer is indicated by a Gleason score of from 8 to 10. It is the most advanced stage of the disease, with poorly differentiated cells that no longer bear a resemblance to the normal cells of the body. No available treatment option can heal this aggressive grade of cancer. Marks notes, "This grade of cancer is rapid-growing, very aggressive and quick to grow into surrounding tissues. They can spread into the lymph nodes and bone."[16] If the cancer has spread outside the gland and into the surrounding tissue and bones, it is less likely that any medical treatment will be able to heal the disease. The focus shifts from curing the cancer to controlling its spread and the pain it may already be causing.

One of the people whose battle with prostate cancer I read about is Benjamin S. Carson Sr., the world-famous neurosurgeon at Johns Hopkins University. He reported that when the pathology report came back, he was diagnosed with high-grade prostate cancer. After he went through a surgical procedure to remove his prostate, he was told that the cancer was only one millimeter away (as close as it could get) from breaking through his prostate gland and spreading to other parts of his body.[17] Ben

Carson is living proof that men can survive even high-grade cancer if they move quickly with an appropriate treatment plan once the diagnosis has been made.

Stages of Prostate Cancer

There is one more step in the diagnosis of prostate cancer that goes along with the grading of the tissue that was taken in the biopsy and the assignment of a Gleason score. This additional step is called *staging*. The staging of prostate cancer is the doctor's evaluation of all the tests that have been done and the determination of how much cancer is in the body and exactly where that cancer is located. In order to accurately determine the stage of the cancer in the body, a doctor may order additional tests, including a bone scan, a biopsy of other potentially impacted tissues of the body, a CT (computed tomography) scan, and in some cases an MRI (magnetic resonance imaging) scan.

It is crucial that you know the stage of your cancer so that you and your doctor can make the best choice about how to proceed with treatment. Grading is different from staging in one clear and significant area. Grading indicates how aggressive the tissue is and how fast it is likely to spread; staging, through the various additional tests, documents just how far, if at all, the cancer has actually spread throughout the prostate and into other parts of the body. As with the Gleason score, the higher the staging number given to your sample tissue, the more aggressive and threatening the cancer is likely to be.[18]

Stages 1 and 2 represent early prostate cancer localized in the prostate gland.

Stage 3 prostate cancer is locally advanced outside the gland.

Stage 4 prostate cancer has spread to other organs or tissues.

If the cancer is limited to only one or two locations in the prostate, that stage is early enough so that many treatment options are available. If the cancer has spread to the point that it can be found on both sides of the prostate, then that stage signals a more advanced condition, with a lower chance of complete healing and an increased chance of long-term side effects. If the cancer is found outside the prostate in the lymph nodes, the bladder, the rectum, or the other organs around the prostate, or if the cancer has moved into the bones, doctors are not inclined to employ the most aggressive treatments for cancer, because they doubt these treatments will have any long-term positive effect.

If you are feeling worried at this point, relax and remember this: most biopsies do not reveal any cancerous tissue at all. Also, let me state again that just because you have an elevated PSA number that leads you to have a biopsy of the prostate, that does not mean that you you will be diagnosed with prostate cancer. I recommended to a clergy colleague of mine here in Cleveland that he go to see my urologist when he was made aware of an elevated PSA score. His biopsy results revealed no cancer in any of the tissue samples.

One report states, "PSA levels that are high enough to trigger suspicion of cancer may be caused simply by other conditions, such as a swollen or irritated prostate. By some estimates, up to 750,000 of the 1 million biopsies performed each year following a suspicious PSA test are unnecessary."[19] I would not have used the word "unnecessary," because it gives the impression that the biopsy did not need to be done. I urge every man with a PSA score above 4 to have a biopsy of his prostate done right away. Some urologists are now suggesting that the biopsy should be done if the PSA score is above 2.5, believing that they would be able to diagnose aggressive cancers at an earlier stage and provide treatment that has a greater chance of a cure.[20] Those same urologists are also suggesting that the age at which all men should start being regularly screened for prostate cancer should be lowered from the age of forty-five or fifty to the age of forty.[21]

You have nothing to lose by taking the precaution of getting a biopsy of the prostate, and you have a great deal to gain. The only thing better than getting an early detection of prostate cancer is to learn that you have no cancer in your body at all.

What Comes Next

This chapter has focused on the issue of what prostate cancer is and how it is detected and then diagnosed. That is the first step in your battle with prostate cancer. The next issue that must be resolved is deciding upon one of the various methods that can be used to treat the stage and grade of cancer that you have developed. Several options are available to you, and your urologist will explain to you the pros and cons of each one. In the next chapter I will attempt to explain what those methods are and why I settled on the treatment plan that was used in my case.

Questions to Consider

♦♦ If you are a man over the age of forty, are you getting an annual physical exam that includes both a digital rectal exam and a PSA blood test?

♦♦ If you are a man over forty years of age, do you know your PSA score?

♦♦ If your PSA score is over 4.0, do you understand the importance of getting a needle biopsy to further determine whether you may have developed prostate cancer?

♦♦ If you have gotten a biopsy, has your urologist given your tissue a Gleason score that measures the stage and grade of your cancer?

♦♦ If you are an African American man over forty years of age, do you realize that you are at the highest risk of contracting prostate cancer and therefore you must be particularly attentive to getting screened for this disease?

✦ Do you know that if your father or your brother has developed prostate cancer, you are now at a higher risk for contracting this disease as well?

✦ Do you know that by the time you begin to feel symptoms related to prostate cancer, the disease may already have advanced to a stage where healing is no longer possible?

✦ Do you know that symptoms of prostate cancer and an elevated PSA score are not guarantees that you have the disease? The biopsy may reveal that you are dealing with some kind of benign problem like a swollen or irritated prostate.

✦ Do you know that prostate cancer is the second most common cancer developed by men, after skin cancer, and that it is the second highest cause of cancer deaths among men, after lung cancer?

✦ Do you know that if prostate cancer is not detected early, while the disease is contained within the prostate gland, it can quickly spread to surrounding tissues, organs, and lymph nodes and into your bones? Early detection of prostate cancer not only increases the number of treatment options available to you, but it also increases the chances that you can be healed of this disease and enjoy a long and healthy life.

Notes

1. American Cancer Society, *Facts on Prostate and Prostate Cancer Testing*, 2002.

2. Sheldon Marks, *Prostate and Cancer: A Family Guide to Diagnosis, Treatment, and Survival* (Cambridge, MA: Fisher, 1999).

3. Patrick Walsh and Janet Farrar Worthington, *Dr. Patrick Walsh's Guide to Surviving Prostate Cancer* (New York: Warner, 2001).

4. Ibid., pp. 21–23.

5. Ibid., pp. 29–30.

6. Ibid., pp. 100–1.

7. Joseph E. Oesterling and Mark A. Moyad, *The ABCs of Prostate Cancer: The Book That Could Save Your Life* (Lanham, MD: Madison, 2003), p. 151.

8. American Cancer Society, *Cancer Facts and Figures, 2003,* pp. 10, 16.

9. American Cancer Society, *Facts on Prostate Cancer,* p. 3.

10. Marks, *Prostate and Cancer,* p. 83.

11. American Cancer Society, *Facts on Prostate Cancer,* p. 4.

12. Dan Fergano, "Improved PSA Test Means Fewer False Positives, Less Controversy," *USA Today,* October 23, 2003, p. D1.

13. Marks, *Prostate and Cancer,* p. 61.

14. Ibid., pp. 78–79.

15. Ibid., p. 83.

16. Ibid., p. 81.

17. Kevin Chappell, "Dr. Ben Carson: Top Surgeon's Life-and-Death Struggle with Prostate Cancer," *Ebony,* January 2003, p. 130.

18. Walsh and Worthington, *Dr. Patrick Walsh's Guide,* pp. 142–43.

19. Vergano, "Improved PSA Test," p. D1.

20. Eric Klein, "Data Support Changing PSA Standards," *Cleveland Clinic Foundation Urology News,* Winter 2003, p. 9.

21. Vergano, "Improved PSA Test," p. D1.

4

Choosing the Right Treatment

Guide my feet, Lord, while I run this race,
'cause I don't want to run this race in vain.
—African American spiritual

THE NEXT STEP IN THE BATTLE WITH PROSTATE CANCER, and perhaps the most decisive step in terms of the medical care that is available to you, involves your decision of how to treat this disease once it has been clinically diagnosed. No single approach to treating prostate cancer applies to every man who develops this disease. How you treat it, and in fact whether you get any treatment at all, depends on several factors, including your age, the stage and grade of your cancer, and your overall physical health.

A man over the age of seventy with an intermediate cancer that is growing slowly may decide not to pursue any aggressive cancer treatment on the grounds that he is likely to die from something else long before his cancer spreads to the point of being life threatening. A man in his fifties with a more aggressive cancer (a Gleason score above 6) may opt for the most aggressive course of treatment in hopes of surviving his cancer and living a normal life span. Your doctor will share with you the pros and cons of the various treatment plans available. There is no one-size-fits-all approach to treating prostate cancer, so ask questions and seek information until you are comfortable about the treatment plan that is best for you and for the stage and grade of cancer you have contracted.

It is crucial for two additional reasons that you clearly understand your options when it comes to choosing a treatment for prostate cancer. The first reason is because of the side effects resulting from certain treatments and the length of the recovery that is required, based on the approach you choose. The second reason you must choose carefully is that some of these treatments can be used together, so if one approach does not remove all of your cancer, another treatment can be used as a follow-up. However, depending on which treatment you use first, you may not be able to take advantage of any of the other methods, and you will then have limited your chances for a complete recovery. Once again, knowledge is power.

There are five standard methods by which prostate cancer is treated, and part of the battle is choosing the one that is right for you. Those five treatment methods are the following:

1. Surgery
2. Radiation therapy
3. Hormone therapy
4. Chemotherapy
5. Watchful waiting[1]

A new treatment for prostate cancer called salvage radiation offers hope to those men who have had a recurrence of an elevated PSA score after they have undergone a radical prostatectomy.

Surgery

Some men may choose to treat their prostate cancer through one of the several available surgical procedures. The most widely known and commonly performed of these surgical procedures is called a *radical prostatectomy*. This is the procedure that my surgeon and I chose for my own cancer treatment.

Radical prostatectomy. This is a procedure in which the entire prostate gland, along with some tissue around that area, is removed. The intent of this operation is to remove the cancer from your body before it has a chance to spread outside the prostate gland and infect other organs and tissue in that area of your body. This is the most aggressive way to treat prostate cancer and offers the best chance for a cure.

There are typically three criteria for deciding who is a good candidate for this procedure.

1. The patient must have prostate cancer that is confined to the prostate.
2. The patient should be able to safely undergo a major operation requiring general anesthesia.
3. The patient should have a life expectancy long enough to see the benefits of this surgery, usually seven to ten years or more.[2]

If you opt for a radical prostatectomy, you must then decide whether you want to use the *perineal* or the *retropubic* approach. The perineal approach involves an incision under the scrotum and in front of the rectum while the legs are elevated. The surgeon must move through layers of tissue and runs the risk of damaging the nerves that control sexual function and bladder control.[3]

The retropubic approach is also called the *nerve-sparing* approach. In this case the incision is made along the abdomen from just below the belly button to the top of the pubic bone. The surgeon gets a much better view of the prostate gland when this method is used, and more importantly for most men, this procedure can be done with minimal impact on the nerves, thus reducing the risk of long-term and perhaps even permanent incontinence and impotence.[4]

No matter which of these two methods you choose, you will likely spend three or four days in the hospital after your surgery, and you will be strongly urged to allow from four to six weeks for a recovery from the surgery before you resume your normal activities. When a radical prostatectomy has been performed, a catheter is inserted, running from the bladder through the penis and into a plastic container called a Foley bag. This allows urine to flow out of the body while the urinary tract recovers from the trauma of the surgery. The catheter remains in place for two or three weeks, though a smaller leg bag is provided so that you can move more freely during the day.

The primary risks attached to this procedure are those of short-term incontinence (loss of bladder control) and impotence (the inability to achieve and maintain an erection). In most cases, men regain control of both these functions as the nerves heal after the operation. There are also a variety of ways by which these functions can be restored if the healing process alone does not restore them fully. However in a small percentage of men, the damage can be long-term and sometimes even permanent.[5]

It is often the fear of these side effects that causes men to avoid getting prostate cancer screening or treating their prostate cancer. I do not want to minimize these side effects, especially as I have had to endure both of them myself even months after the surgery. However, I know of prostate cancer survivors who suffered no incontinence at all and whose struggle with impotence was short-lived. These are *possible* side effects, and that means they will not occur in every case. Furthermore, men will experience these side effects for different periods of time and to different degrees.

On the other hand, the only reason to have a radical prostatectomy is to remove an aggressive cancer that is present inside of your body. Ignoring that reality simply to avoid temporary incontinence or impotence is gambling with your life. Bladder control and sexual function can be restored in the vast majority of cases, but if you do not act quickly and the cancer in your prostate gland spreads to other organs and tissues in your body, then bladder control and sexual function will be the least of your concerns. Untreated prostate cancer can kill you. It is essential that you not allow your anxieties about the side effects of this surgery to prevent you from taking action that can save your life. Early detection and swift and appropriate treatment are the keys to surviving prostate cancer, and a radical prostatectomy is one of those treatment methods.

Other surgical procedures. Along with the usual type of radical prostatectomy, doctors sometimes recommend a new and less invasive form of prostate surgery known as the *laparoscopic radical prostatectomy*. This involves "the use of a lighted tube that enters the body through a tiny hole through which a surgeon can thread a scalpel.... There is a smaller incision, fewer side effects and a shorter recovery time."[6]

Another procedure is known as *cryosurgery*, which involves inserting a metal probe directly into the cancerous tissue and trying to destroy the cancerous cells by freezing them with liquid nitrogen.[7] Cryosurgery is still in the experimental stages and its long-term results are not known. This procedure creates similar side effects to the more usual kinds of surgery, and there remains the possibility that the cancer may return, since the prostate gland itself is not removed during this procedure.

Check with your urologist to determine if either of these newer procedures may be right for you.

Radiation Therapy

Another way of treating prostate cancer that does not require surgery and anesthesia, and that does not require a long hospital stay and an even longer period of recuperation, is radiation therapy. This form of therapy uses high-energy rays or particles to kill cancer cells. This involves one of two approaches to delivering radiation to the cancerous tissue. One method is called *external beam radiation therapy*, in which beams of high-intensity radiation are directed from outside the body onto the target area where cancerous tissue has been discovered. The other method of delivery is called *internal radiation therapy* or *brachytherapy*, in which radioactive pellets the size of a grain of rice are implanted into the cancerous areas of the prostate so that the radioactivity can work from within the body to kill the cancer.

External beam radiation therapy. The external beam approach to radiation therapy involves going for radiation treatment every day from Monday to Friday for six or seven weeks. The treatments take from ten to fifteen minutes to administer, and treatment typically is not given on weekends so that the normal cells in the body can recover from the high doses of radiation that are used to kill the cancerous cells. The primary goal of external beam radiation therapy is to control the growth and spread of cancer cells without going through the trauma of a surgical procedure.[8]

Internal radiation therapy, or brachytherapy. This process uses a needle to insert radioactive seeds the size of a grain of rice directly into predetermined locations within the prostate gland. The seeds emit enough radiation to kill any cancerous cells in that area. While this procedure is performed under one of various types of anesthesia that are available, men often return home the same day or may spend just one night in the hospital. Unlike external beam radiation, in which multiple treatments are required, brachytherapy is a one-time procedure. The seeds that are inserted remain effective within the prostate gland for up to several months.

The best candidates for the seed implant procedure are older men with low-grade cancers and a PSA score under 10 and a Gleason score under 7. For this procedure to be effective, it is also essential that the cancer be contained within the prostate gland.

If the cancer has spread to other parts of the body, neither of these radiation therapies will be effective.[9]

Radiation therapy in either of these forms remains a more conservative approach to treating prostate cancer than a radical prostatectomy, primarily because it does not remove the prostate gland. This means there is always the possibility that the cancer can reappear in the prostate—somewhere that was not impacted by the radiation. Moreover, while this procedure keeps you from undergoing a surgical procedure and from facing a long recovery time, it places you at risk for the same side effects as if the surgery had been performed. The most notable of those side effects are temporary incontinence and impotence.

Hormone Therapy

For men whose cancer has already spread beyond the prostate to other parts of the body, hormone therapy may be the best treatment. The goal of hormone therapy is to decrease the amount of the male hormone called *testosterone* that is produced by a man's body. Testosterone is produced mainly inside the testicles and can allow prostate cancer cells to grow. By reducing the testosterone levels in the body, you can make prostate cancer shrink, or grow more slowly. Thus hormone therapy should be viewed as a way to control the spread of, but not to cure, prostate cancer.[10]

In some cases your doctor may recommend the surgical removal of the testicles as a way to reduce testosterone. This procedure is called an *orchiectomy*.[11] Obviously some men will be reluctant to go through this procedure, which is synonymous with being castrated. The testicles are surgically removed from the scrotum. Remember, however, that with advanced-stage prostate cancer that has spread outside of the gland to other parts of the body, this aggressive treatment might prolong your life considerably.

For those who choose not to reduce their testosterone level through this surgical procedure, there is another way to proceed; it is called *injection therapy*. This involves receiving injections of hormone medications into either the buttocks or the lower abdominal wall. The injections are initially given on a monthly basis; however, once it has been determined that you can tolerate this medicine, your doctor may switch you to an injection that is effective for three or four months at a time.[12] If you opt for hormone therapy, you will have to receive these injections on a regular basis (every month or every three to four months) for the rest of your life.

Chemotherapy

When prostate cancer has spread outside the prostate gland, and when hormone therapy has not been successful in slowing down the spread of the disease, chemotherapy is a final treatment option. Chemotherapy involves the use of drugs to kill cancer cells, slow the growth of cancerous tumors, and reduce the pain that comes with high-grade, aggressive prostate cancer that has spread outside the prostate gland.

Chemotherapy involves either taking a pill or receiving the drug intravenously through a needle. The drug flows through the bloodstream and kills cancer cells throughout the body. These are powerful drugs, and the downside of chemotherapy for any kind of cancer treatment is that it also kills normal cells in the body. Like hormone therapy, chemotherapy does not offer any prospect of curing your prostate cancer. It should be viewed solely as an attempt to slow its growth and control the pain.

Dr. Sheldon Marks offers a candid assessment of this method of treating prostate cancer when he says, "The big question with chemotherapy is whether its possible benefits outweigh its probable side effects. The treatment may add only a few months to your life span, and you may spend those months weak and nauseated."[13] The side effects can also include vomiting, hair loss, and even heart problems.[14]

Watchful Waiting

For two groups of men, the best response to prostate cancer may be to do nothing right away. For younger men (seventy years of age or less) with cancer that is contained within only one area of the prostate and that is growing very slowly, their doctor may suggest that they just wait a while and see how things develop over time. For elderly men who have additional health problems, the watch-and-wait approach may also be preferred. Prostate cancer spreads very slowly, and among older men there is a chance they will die from either natural causes or other medical complications.[15]

Another term for watchful waiting is *expectant management.* This implies that while younger men may not be taking any aggressive action in terms of treating prostate cancer, they are taking some precautionary measures. These include closely monitoring their PSA level, getting occasional digital rectal exams, and possibly getting a urinalysis to be sure their condition is not changing for the worse. If a patient begins to notice a rise in his PSA level or starts seeing blood in his urine, then he should be concerned and should consider starting one of the treatments for prostate cancer.

The central issue is this: If a man and his doctor decide that any aggressive treatment and the side effects that will follow are more severe than any benefit he is likely to experience from that treatment, he may want to try watchful waiting.[16]

If you do choose watching waiting as your initial approach to treatment, however, be sure that you *are* watching with care because prostate cancer is a silent and stealthy attacker which cannot be ignored.

New Treatments for Prostate Cancer

A new treatment for prostate cancer called *salvage radiation* was announced in the March 2004 issue of the *Journal of the American Medical Association*. Salvage radiation offers hope to those men who have had a recurrence of an elevated PSA score after they have undergone a radical prostatectomy. A study was done at the Baylor College of Medicine in Houston, Texas, involving 501 men whose PSA scores rose within ten months of their surgery. Prior to this study, it was believed that an elevated PSA score not only indicated that cancer had returned, but that it had probably spread to other parts of the body.[17]

In those instances, doctors had traditionally treated men only with hormone therapy to slow the growth of the cancer, believing that radiation designed to eliminate the cancer would not work. This new study found that fifty percent of the men who fit into this category and were treated with this form of radiation therapy remained cancer-free an average of four years later. Dr. Kevin Slawin, the lead author for the study said, "Salvage radiation changed the natural history of that disease."[18] Not only is this study good news for the men who fall within this category of cancer patients, but it also keeps hope alive that researchers will continue to find new treatments and cures for all of the men who are fighting their own battle with prostate cancer.

NOTES

1. American Cancer Society, *Facts on Prostate Cancer and Prostate Cancer Testing*, 2002, pp. 6–9.
2. Sheldon Marks, *Prostate and Cancer: A Family Guide to Diagnosis, Treatment, and Survival* (Cambridge, MA: Fisher, 1999), p. 159.
3. Patrick Walsh and Janet Farrar Worthington, *Dr. Patrick Walsh's Guide to Surviving Prostate Cancer* (New York: Warner, 2001), p. 238.

4. Ibid., p. 223.

5. Marks, *Prostate and Cancer*, pp. 223–44.

6. Walsh and Worthington, *Dr. Patrick Walsh's Guide*, p. 239.

7. Marks, *Prostate and Cancer*, pp. 214–17.

8. Walsh and Worthington, *Dr. Patrick Walsh's Guide*, pp. 259–69.

9. Ibid., pp. 270–81.

10. Marks, *Prostate and Cancer*, pp. 196–213.

11. Joseph E. Oesterling and Mark A. Moyad, *The ABCs of Prostate Cancer: The Book That Could Save Your Life* (Lanham, MD: Madison, 2003), pp. 152–54.

12. Marks, *Prostate and Cancer*, pp. 206–8.

13. Ibid., p. 277.

14. American Cancer Society, *Facts on Prostate Cancer*, p. 9.

15. Marks, *Prostate and Cancer*, pp. 118–21.

16. Oesterling and Moyad, *ABCs of Prostate Cancer*, pp. 105–8.

17. Lindsey Tanner, "Study Suggests Radiation as Prostate Cancer Cure," *The Plain Dealer*, March 17, 2004, p. A11.

18. Ibid.

5

Facing Treatment with Faith

Even though I walk
through the valley of the shadow of death,
I will fear no evil,
for you are with me.
—Psalm 23:4, NIV

ONE OF THE MOST OFTEN QUOTED LINES IN AMERICAN
political history was written by Thomas Paine, an American
patriot of the Revolutionary War. In the winter of 1776 he wrote
an essay entitled "The American Crisis" that was meant to challenge and encourage the people who had recently declared their
independence from England. On July 4, 1776, the Declaration of
Independence was signed in Philadelphia, the former colonies
declaring their intention to live as a free and independent nation
with no further ties to the British Empire. However, in the
months that followed, the American patriots discovered that the
forces of Great Britain had no intention of simply sailing away
across the Atlantic Ocean. The British government intended to
press its claim and force the American colonies back into their
prior position as subjects of the crown.

In those five months from July to December of 1776, many of
the people who had initially been enthusiastic about the
prospects of independence began to lose their fervor. They began
to abandon the cause of freedom and fall back in line with the

British. The infant revolution was on the verge of collapse before it had really begun. It was into that climate that Thomas Paine directed words that most of us remember from elementary school. He wrote:

> These are the times that try men's souls. The summer soldier and the sunshine patriot will, in this crisis, shrink from the service of his country; but he that stands it NOW, deserves the love and thanks of man and woman. Tyranny, like hell, is not easily conquered; yet we have this consolation with us, that the harder the conflict, the more glorious the triumph, what we obtain too cheap, we esteem too lightly.[1]

Thomas Paine was telling his fellow Americans something of great importance. The mark of our character and the depth of our commitment are not measured by how we perform when life is good and everything comes easily into our reach. Rather, the true measure of our souls is best determined by how we respond when the going gets tough and every forward step seems like a struggle. Those, indeed, are the times that try men's souls.

The message from that eighteenth-century American patriot is no less compelling in the twenty-first century as you and I try to navigate our way through the challenges and setbacks that confront us every day. And the words are applicable not only in a political setting but work just as well in the professional, personal, physical, financial, and emotional issues that may be confronting us right now. If you have ever been confronted with a diagnosis of cancer that has challenged your faith or shattered your peace or obscured your vision of the future, then let me build upon the words of Thomas Paine: These are the times that try men's souls. Summer Christians and sunshine disciples will not be able to stand the test. But remember that the harder the conflict, the more glorious the victory.

The Tool of Faith

The apostle Paul seems to have understood this issue long before Thomas Paine wrote his famous essay. In Philippians 4:12-13, Paul declared that he was not someone who would serve the cause of Jesus Christ only when everything was going his way. He was not a summer Christian or a sunshine disciple. Paul declared, "I know how to be abased and I know how to abound. I know how to be empty and I know how to be full. I can do all things through Christ who strengthens me."

Not every day of life will be easy, yet we, too, can do all things through Christ who strengthens us. We may be riding high today and be brought low tomorrow, but we can do all things through Christ who strengthens us. We may in the best of health when we wake up in the morning and end up in the hospital before the sun goes down on that same day. The future may look like a steep, uphill journey with pitfalls on every side. You may be facing a cancer surgery, a battery of chemotherapy or radiation treatments; or the sad news that a condition long in remission has returned with even greater and more damaging effect. The power and promise of this text from Philippians is what all of us must cling to every day: I can do all things through Christ who strengthens me!

Recognition by Medical Science

The November 10, 2003, issue of *Newsweek* magazine made the point that many people in the medical field now affirm that faith in God during times of sickness greatly contributes to a patient's rate of recovery. While not all medical professionals agree, there seems to be a growing number of doctors and nurses who view religious faith, especially in the form of prayer, as a source of comfort and assurance for patients who are facing serious illness. In this regard, medical science is catching up with a view widely held throughout American society, where 84 percent of the people polled for that article believe that praying for the sick improves their chances of recovery.[2]

Dr. Harold Koenig of Duke University, a pioneer in the research concerning faith and medicine, points to a growing body of evidence of religion's positive effect upon health. Koenig states, "Keeping spirituality out of the clinic is irresponsible." He notes that "patient after patient tells me that religion is the most important thing; it keeps them going."[3]

Koenig is not alone in his conviction that religious faith is a factor in how people cope with their sickness. More than 70 of the nation's 125 medical schools now offer courses dealing with faith and healing, or they incorporate that topic into the curriculum in other ways.

Paul was speaking even for those of us who have been battling prostate cancer when he said, "I can do all things through Christ who strengthens me." The strength and depth of your faith in God can make an enormous difference as you try to cope with the diagnosis, treatment, and survival of prostate cancer.

The Changeable Circumstances of Life

I would not be surprised if the announcement that you have contracted prostate cancer caught you by surprise. That certainly was true in my case. The premise of the statements by Paul and by Thomas Paine is that the conditions and circumstances of our lives, and of the lives of those around us, can change quickly. The world as we know it today may look very different tomorrow.

I recently received an e-mail from a young minister who earned the Ph.D. degree from Harvard University. He was establishing himself as a leader within the theological community, writing highly regarded books and scholarly essays. Both he and his wife had secured teaching positions at a seminary in

Texas. There seemed to be no limit to where my friend's career would take him.

Then in February of this year, while he and his wife were turning into the driveway of their home in Texas, their subcompact car was hit and demolished by a speeding SUV. His wife suffered serious spinal damage, from which she has partially recovered. My friend was not so lucky. His injuries were so severe that the hip replacements he had already received were destroyed, and he is now permanently confined to a wheelchair. He cannot walk even with crutches. In a moment, their whole world was turned upside down.

Let me say again that the conditions and circumstances of your life today are not guaranteed to remain that way tomorrow. If nothing has challenged your life yet, just keep living and you, too, will come to moments described by Thomas Paine as "the times that try men's souls." The question for today is, what will you do when such a day comes? Will you commit suicide because you cannot imagine living in a world that is not perfect every day? Will you throw yourself a "pity party" and tell God that you do not deserve what has happened to you? I hope you will respond as Paul has suggested in this passage, saying, "I know how to be abased and I know how to abound. I know how to be empty and I know how to be full. I can do all things through Christ who strengthens me."

Lest we forget what Paul had to endure during his life and ministry, let's revisit his testimony in 2 Corinthians 11:24-25. He reminds us that five times he was beaten with thirty-nine lashes, three times he was beaten with sticks, once he was stoned, three times he was shipwrecked, and once he spent an entire day and night adrift in the waters of the Mediterranean Sea. Paul says that his life was punctuated by sufferings, hardships, setbacks, dangers, and perils. Yet he endured in the face of all of that, and in our passage in Philippians he tells us the secret of his ability to persevere.

Paul says, "I can do all things through Christ who strengthens me."

Let me encourage you to lay claim to this passage and to this promise from God. It is possible for us to hold on and persevere in whatever condition we find ourselves, so long as we hold onto our faith in God.

Look around you and be reminded of how many lives are suddenly turned upside down. People are losing their jobs. Marriages are coming apart at the seams. Death has robbed people of their loved ones. Sons and daughters are fighting in wars all over the world.

What can be said to people who are trying to hold on in the face of these challenging circumstances? May I suggest, first of all, the paraphrased words of Thomas Paine? This is no time to be a summer Christian or a sunshine disciple. These are the times that try men's souls. My second suggestion would be to lay claim to the paraphrased words of Paul—Christ can give you the strength to endure and overcome anything life throws your way.

Remember that the strength is not yours; it comes from Christ. And when you come through your crisis, the glory will not be yours but will belong to Christ. Here is the gospel message for today, here is the good news from God: you can do all things through Christ who strengthens you.

Faith on Trial

In his book *The Lord's Prayer: In Times Such as These,* Frank Thomas reminds us that the phrase "lead us not into temptation" can also be read as "lead us not into trials or tests."[4] The Greek word *peirasmos* carries that double meaning. Thomas goes on to remind us that trials or tests, such as contracting cancer, losing a job, going through an unhappy divorce proceeding, or enduring the tragic and untimely death of a loved one, are tests of our character and trials of our faith in God. He says, "Trials have to do with different situations we find ourselves in that test and measure our confidence in God."[5] In fact, says Thomas, "A trial is something we would rather avoid."

> We don't want our confidence in God tested. We don't want our earth shaken up. We don't want our world rearranged. We don't want our set agenda, our career plans all messed up. A trial is something that we would rather avoid. A trial is a challenge to test what we are made of and ultimately to see what we believe.[6]

Has this happened in your life? Has your cancer diagnosis tested your confidence in God? That was initially true for me, and I would not be surprised if it is true for any person who believes in God. The question is not only "Why has God allowed this to happen to me?" but also "Is God able to bring me through this critical time in my life?" It is perfectly natural for these questions and concerns to rush into your mind when you have just been diagnosed with cancer; that is the moment when your faith in God really goes on trial. The challenge is to move from questioning God because of what has happened and to start laying claim to all that God has promised to do for God's people in times such as these.

Andraé Crouch wrote a song entitled "Through It All" in which the following lines appear: "Through it all,... I learned to trust in Jesus, I learned to trust in God."[7] Well, I invite you to trust in two passages from God's Word as you are dealing with the diagnosis, treatment, and recovery period of your battle with cancer. They are Romans 5:1-5 and James 1:2-4. Both of these passages carry the message that the physical and spiritual test you are undergoing can make you stronger than you were before.

The Romans 5 passage says, "Suffering produces perseverance, and perseverance produces character, and character produces hope, and hope does not disappoint us." We can come through the experience of prostate cancer. We can endure the shock, disbelief, uncertainty, medical procedures, and long-term recovery that are involved in this process. The same God who has sustained us through all of life's earlier trials and tests is able to do it again. The hope with which we face the future is grounded in our recollection of all our former times of trial when God proved trustworthy to sustain us and bring us safely through.

The passage in James invites us to see our present sickness or suffering as an opportunity for God to do a great work in our lives. That passage says, "Consider it pure joy, my brothers, whenever you face trials of many kinds, because you know that the testing of your faith develops perseverance. Perseverance must finish its work so that you may be mature and complete, not lacking anything" (James 1:2-4, NIV).

J. Alfred Smith offers a comment on this passage in *The African American Devotional Bible*. He mentions how J. B. Phillips restates the verse by saying, "When all kinds of trials and temptations crowd into your lives, my brothers, don't resent them as intruders, but welcome them as friends. Realize that they come to test your faith and to produce in you the quality of endurance."[8] Smith then goes on to observe this:

> How strange it seems to call suffering a friend when it gives us heartbreak and heartache. But James suggests that the purpose of suffering is to help, not to hurt. You and I are called to look past immediate hurt to see long-range good. What is this long-range good? It is the maturation of our faith.[9]

The Roots of Faith

As news began to spread across the city of Cleveland about the cancer surgery that I would soon be facing, someone from outside my congregation sent me a Hallmark card with an anonymous verse entitled "The Oak Tree," which greatly encouraged me.

Now I share its message with others who are entering the battle with prostate cancer or any other similar challenge.

The verse spoke of a giant oak tree that was battered by howling winds until all of its leaves had been stripped off and most of its bark had been torn away. But the oak tree had roots that stretched deep into the earth, and it was those deep roots that kept the tree standing in the face of the fierce winds that blew so hard against it.

That can and should be the testimony of every Christian. Let the winds wail and roar all around us, and let the harsh realities of life rip at our limbs and branches and outer bark. We can stand in the face of that torment if we have sunk our roots deep in God and allow God to hold us up when the world tries to blow us down. In fact, we do not know how strong we are or how much we can endure until we spend some time in a storm, and only then will we know for sure that our roots can hold us secure when the storms of life are raging.

That was the word of assurance and comfort about which David wrote in Psalm 23. Life can find us in green pastures and beside still waters one day, and suddenly we can be plunged into the valley of the shadow of death. That is no time or place for a "sunshine Christian." That is the time to lean on your faith and make your way through that perilous place, not because you are relying upon your own strength, but because God will be with you.

Once you are diagnosed with prostate cancer, as I was, you do not have to panic. I came through the diagnosis, the treatment, and many of the follow-up procedures that are often a part of the postoperation recovery and healing process. Today my PSA level is undetectable. I am living as a *cancer survivor.* I am living *cancer free.* My faith has sustained me throughout this yearlong ordeal, and your faith can and will do the same for you.

We can do all things through Christ who strengthens us.

NOTES

1. Thomas Paine, "The American Crisis," in *The American Reader: Words That Moved a Nation,* edited by Diane Ravitch (New York: Harper-Collins, 1990), p. 28.

2. Claudia Kalb, "Faith and Healing," *Newsweek,* November 10, 2003, p. 46.

3. Quoted in ibid., pp. 47, 53.

4. Frank A. Thomas, *The Lord's Prayer: In Times Such as These* (St. Louis: Chalice, 2002), p. 75.

5. Ibid., p. 77.

6. Ibid., pp. 77–78.

7. Andraé Crouch, "Through It All," *The Best of Lift Him Up* (Nashville: Benson, 1994), pp. 133–34.

8. J. Alfred Smith, "Commentary on James 1:2-4," in *The African American Devotional Bible* (Grand Rapids, MI: Zondervan, 1997), p. 1389.

9. Ibid.

6

Reducing the Risk of Prostate Cancer

Dear friend, I pray that you may enjoy good health and that all may go well with you, even as your soul is getting along well.
—3 John 2, NIV

UP TO THIS POINT, THIS BOOK HAS ADDRESSED THE CHAL-lenge of responding to a diagnosis of prostate cancer. But now I want to take a step back and discuss how this disease might be prevented. One of the first thoughts that crossed my mind after I was diagnosed with prostate cancer was to wonder what I might have done differently earlier in my life to keep me from con-tracting this disease. Unfortunately, I never stopped to consider how cancer could be prevented until it had already developed within my body to the point that treatment was needed. In the months since my surgery, I have read every book and article I could find that deals with preventing, or at least reducing the risk of developing, prostate cancer. What I have discovered is that I could have taken some steps that would have greatly reduced my chances of developing this disease or could at least have slowed down the spread of the cancer so that the surgical treatment I underwent might not have been needed so soon.

This chapter obviously comes much too late to be of any ben-efit to me so far as prostate cancer prevention is concerned. How-ever, it is my earnest and sincere hope that what I have learned about cancer prevention can and will be of great help to other men. The only thing better than detecting cancer early is not developing cancer at all.

You are not powerless. There are some things you can do to reduce your risk of developing prostate cancer.

Four Risk Factors

In considering how to prevent or reduce your risk of developing prostate cancer, you need to begin by determining whether you fit into one of the four groups of men who are most at risk for this disease. The categories are influenced by the following characteristics:

- Age
- Race or ethnicity
- Environment
- Family history

Based on these categories, if you are a man who faces an increased risk for developing prostate cancer, you need to be particularly aggressive in taking steps to lower that risk as much as possible.

1. Age. Prostate cancer is a disease that affects men as they get older. It is rarely seen in men who are in their twenties and thirties. It is recommended, therefore, that men begin being screened for the disease when they enter their forties. Signs of the disease begin to show up more frequently, either in the digital rectal exam or the PSA blood test, when men enter their fifties. Dr. Joseph Oesterling says, "By age 50, almost 33 percent of men have small prostate tumors. By age 80 about 75 percent of men are believed to have prostate cancer, and by age 90, about 90 percent have the disease."[1] This confirms the common perception that prostate cancer is of greatest concern for older men. However, bear in mind that I was diagnosed and treated for this disease at the age of fifty-four.

2. Race/Ethnicity. Your racial or ethnic background plays a significant role in determining whether you are at higher for prostate cancer. All of the data suggest that African Americans are about twice as likely to develop this disease as any other racial group in the world. In fact, African American men "seem to get more severe forms of prostate cancer, are more likely to have cancer recur after treatment, and are more likely to die from the disease than white men."[2] The lowest incidences of prostate cancer are found among Asians, notably men from China and Japan. The following graph suggests how prostate cancer impacts various racial groups around the world.

Race and Ethnicity:	Percentage of deaths due to prostate cancer:
Blacks	9.4%
Whites	6.3%
Native Americans	5.9%
Hispanics	5.7%
Asians and Pacific Islanders	3.9%[3]

While medical scientists are not sure why African Americans seem to be at a greater risk for developing prostate cancer, one of the reasons the disease is so lethal within that population may have something to do with typical male behaviors that need to be confronted and altered. Most men (black, white, and every shade in between) are reluctant to undergo the digital rectal exam. They resist the idea of having someone probing inside their rectum.

Add to the universal dislike of DRE the additional tendency among many African American men not to seek medical advice and treatment for this disease until they are already experiencing painful symptoms. That means that the cancer has probably already spread outside the prostate gland, and in those instances the chances of being cured are greatly reduced; the most that doctors and medicines can do is slow the growth of the cancer and control the pain it causes. It is essential, then, that African American men, who are already at greater risk for developing prostate cancer, be aggressive in reducing their risk by seeing a doctor regularly and by being screened for prostate cancer with the DRE and the PSA test.

As a purely economic factor, some men may not be seeing a doctor because they do not have any medical insurance and do not qualify either for Medicare or Medicaid. The fact that we have the finest health care system in the world is a matter of great pride for the United States. The fact that 45 million of our fellow citizens have little or no medical insurance is a fact that should cause us great shame.

We can quickly find $87 billion to rebuild Iraq after we destroyed that country in a war whose purpose is less than clear and whose outcome is less than certain. We can suddenly find billions of dollars to extend the space exploration program with talk of landing an astronaut on Mars. At the same time, however, we cannot make our wonderful medical system available to 45 million of our own people.

3. Environment. One of the things that is not widely known about reducing the risk for prostate cancer is the positive effect of regular but moderate exposure to sunshine and the ultraviolet rays it produces. While overexposure can result in skin cancer, science and medicine agree that moderate exposure to ultraviolet radiation "has a protective effect against prostate cancer. It seems that ultraviolet radiation activates the production of vitamin D in the body, and vitamin D is known to have some anti-cancer effects."[4]

This helps to explain why prostate cancer deaths are highest among men who live in places like Scandinavia, Western Europe, and North America, which have lower amounts of sunshine over the course of a year and thus are exposed to lower amounts of ultraviolet radiation. This also helps to explain why men living in the northern part of the United States have a higher incidence of prostate cancer than men living in the southern United States, where there is a higher exposure to sunlight during the year.[5]

This may also help to explain why black men are twice as likely to develop prostate cancer, because the darker pigment of their skin absorbs less ultraviolet radiation and thus their bodies naturally produce less vitamin D. One study done by African scientists highlights the influence of exposure even among dark-skinned men, however. The study compared blood levels of vitamin D in black men living in Zaire (now the Democratic Republic of the Congo) with Zairian black men living in Belgium (the former colonial ruler of that African nation). There was a significantly lower level of vitamin D in the black men living in Western Europe as compared to the higher levels found in those black men who lived in the sunnier climate of Central Africa.[6]

There is a measurable benefit to having regular, moderate exposure to sunshine and the vitamin D that it produces. Of course, one can get the benefits of vitamin D through a diet that includes a moderate amount of dairy products. However, you need to be careful not to overconsume dairy products and the high-fat content found in such food products as whole milk, butter, ice cream, and certain cheeses. Check with your physician to determine the safest way for you to access the cancer-preventive benefits of vitamin D.

4. Family history. If a member of your family has had this disease, you are at a higher risk of developing the disease yourself. The greater the number of family members who have had the disease, the higher is your risk not only of getting prostate cancer but also of developing it at an earlier age. Be sure to inquire on both sides of your family (men on your father's and mother's sides of the family) to see if any of them have been diagnosed with this disease.

If a man in your family has been diagnosed with prostate cancer, "then that man's sons, brothers, cousins and nephews should start being seen yearly for the PSA exam beginning at age 40, and should make preventive dietary changes now."[7] If you have been diagnosed with prostate cancer, then you need to encourage the other men in your family to be screened when they turn forty years of age, and you need to advise them to substantially alter their diet to help reduce their risk of developing cancer.

One of the things that I now have bequeathed to my son is an increased risk of developing this disease. We talked about that when I shared the news with him about my diagnosis, and while he is only twenty-three years old right now, he will have to pay close attention to this aspect of his health as he gets older. And as mentioned above, he needs to alter his diet now as one way to lower his risk of developing the disease that threatened his father's life.

I now wonder if any man in my family ever had prostate cancer and if I developed it as a result of my own family history. My father did die of cancer at the age of eighty-one, but since he had been a long-time cigarette smoker and had been a house painter who was always inhaling fumes from paint and turpentine, I always assumed that the cause of his death was lung cancer. It did not occur to me until after I was diagnosed that he might also have had prostate cancer. Once again it must be underscored that when men remain quiet about the fact that they have developed prostate cancer, they are doing a disservice to every younger male member of their family, which includes sons, cousins, nephews, and brothers.

One man's silence about his battle with prostate cancer can result in another man having to fight that same battle years later. The sooner a man diagnosed with prostate cancer shares the news, the sooner the younger men in his family can start taking steps to lower their risk of developing this disease. As mentioned above, the steps that can be taken are, first of all, being screened beginning at the age of forty and, second, making preventive dietary changes.[8]

The Impact of Diet

Every major study ever done on the prevention of prostate cancer has agreed that the foods we eat greatly impact our risk of developing this disease. Men who eat a high-fat diet that includes a lot of red meat and dairy products have an increased risk of developing prostate cancer. Conversely, men who maintain a low-fat diet that includes an ample amount of fresh fruits, soy-based products, and other vegetables, especially tomatoes and tomato-based products, can substantially lower their risk of developing this disease.

What first alerted cancer researchers to the importance of diet was the experience of Asian men who fit into two separate categories. Asian men, especially those living in China and Japan, have the lowest incidences of prostate cancer of any men in the world. However, when men born in Asia move out of that region and spend at least twenty-five years living in the West, either the United States or Western Europe, their rate of developing prostate cancer greatly increases. What is even more revealing is the fact that their sons and grandsons develop prostate cancer at the same rate as any other group of men living in the West.[9]

What causes this dramatic increase in the incidences of prostate cancer among Asian men now living in the West? Medical science suggests that the answer involves a change from the low-fat diet common in most places in Asia to the high-fat diet, especially a diet rich in red meat and dairy products, that is so prevalent in Western Europe and the United States.[10]

Dr. Patrick Walsh notes that diet impacts the fight against prostate cancer in one of two ways: either prevention of the disease or a slowing of the growth of cancer that has already begun. He says,

How can your diet help your body fight prostate cancer? There are two main ways: The first is in preventing or delaying the onset of the disease. Cancer that is big enough to be diagnosed today probably started growing at least ten years ago. Most men are diagnosed with prostate cancer in their late sixties. This means that even men in their fifties and early sixties should be able to make a significant difference in their body's ability to fight off cancer.[11]

This is a tip about prostate cancer prevention. The diet we follow in our twenties, thirties, and forties can greatly impact our risk of getting this disease. We should not wait until we have been diagnosed to ask, "What could I have done to prevent this disease?" We should act earlier in life and try to prevent getting cancer.

Walsh goes on to note:

The second area of promise is in slowing the growth of cancer that has already begun. Here, diet is one of several avenues being explored to lengthen the life of a man with established or advanced prostate cancer—with the ultimate goal of managing it as a chronic disease, like diabetes or even AIDS, which may not be possible to cure, but which can be controlled for many years.[12]

The question is, what diet should a man follow if he wants to prevent or slow the growth of prostate cancer? Here is what both medical science and the American Cancer Society suggest.

Ideally, the goal should be a Mediterranean diet—one that is high in garlic, tomatoes, red wine and fresh fruits and vegetables, low in beef and dairy products. In addition, a rural Japanese diet is considered healthful—high in fresh vegetables, minimal meat, plenty of soy and green tea.[13]

More precisely, says Patrick Walsh,

Make sure most of what you eat comes from plants. Eat five or more servings of fruits and vegetables a day, and other foods from plant sources, including breads, grains, rice, pasta, or beans, several times a day. Eat foods low in fat, and limit your consumption of meats high in fat.[14]

Most likely you have heard this information before. I was in elementary school when I first heard the rhyme "An apple a day keeps the doctor away." But somehow I always chose apple pie over an apple. The fact is that my doctor has been urging me to alter my diet for years, and everything he has told me has been reinforced by magazine articles and by segments of the evening news. However, it seems that no sooner has the news story about eating a healthier diet gone off the air than it is followed by a commercial advertising fried chicken, a double cheeseburger, or a thick steak with potatoes and gravy. The high-fat American diet is hard to avoid and hard to resist.

It seems that persuading Americans to change their diet is easier said than done. Despite all the warnings about clogged arteries, diabetes, high blood pressure, and obesity, and now despite the clear links between diet and cancer, Americans continue to adhere to a high-fat diet that includes a lot of red meat and not nearly enough fresh fruits and vegetables.

It should be added that a change in diet can even benefit men who have had their prostate removed, as I have. The foods that are useful in preventing prostate cancer are also good for reducing our risk of contracting other types of cancer as well as for reducing our risk of heart disease, stroke, and many other health problems.

What is needed is not just a change in diet but also a substantial change in lifestyle. A recent editorial in an American medical journal stated, "Cancer is largely a preventable illness. Two thirds of cancer deaths in the U.S. can be linked to tobacco use, poor diet, obesity, and lack of exercise, all of which can be modified."[15] Add to these facts this additional observation: the risk of getting prostate cancer rises with the amount of alcohol consumed. According to a recent study, "men who have 22 or more alcoholic drinks per week increase their risk of getting prostate cancer."[16]

I have not smoked cigarettes for over thirty years, and I have never abused alcoholic beverages. However, I am an African American male who has maintained a high-fat diet, never eaten a consistently high amount of fresh fruits or vegetables, specifically avoided tomatoes for most of my life, carried too much body weight, lived a basically sedentary lifestyle for the last ten years of my adult life, and lived in a northern city where the sky is overcast more than 220 days a year. My father died of some type of cancer. When I think about how I have lived my life in light of what I now know about the prevention of prostate cancer, I am not at all surprised that I developed this disease. I now spend a lot of time saying to myself, "If I only knew then what I know now."

What are the foods we should be incorporating into a healthy diet?

Tomatoes. The one thing many researchers agree upon that may lower the risk or slow the spread of prostate cancer is eating a diet that is high in tomatoes and in tomato-based products, such as tomato sauce, pizza, ketchup, and spaghetti. Consuming ten or more servings of tomato-based products per week reduces the risk of contracting prostate cancer by as much as 35 percent. This is because of a vitamin-like substance in tomatoes known as lycopene that helps prevent damage to DNA and that may help lower protaste cancer risk. Lycopene is also found in other fruits and vegetables that are rich in color, such as red peppers, pink grapefruit, strawberries, watermelon, and guava.

It is important to note that as men get older, the amount of lycopene stored in their body decreases, making it necessary that they consume more of the foods that provide this important nutrient. Lycopene is not only effective in reducing the risk of prostate cancer; it also reduces the risk of cancer of the stomach, lungs, breast, bladder, and skin and of leukemia.

For most of my life I avoided eating tomatoes. If they were served as part of a meal, I would always leave them on the plate. If I were eating at a buffet, I would never select tomatoes, even as part of my salad. I would prepare a salad by piling cheese and strips or chunks of meat on top of my lettuce. I would also try to squeeze in some macaroni salad or potato salad that was soaked in mayonnaise. Then I would smother all of that in a high-fat, creamy salad dressing. However, I would intentionally avoid the tomatoes or green peppers that carried the nutrients I needed the most. I have only recently developed a taste for tomatoes, and while this change cannot help me with the prevention of prostate cancer, it can help to reduce my risk of developing other medical conditions that are equally as life threatening.

The "Mediterranean diet." We have already heard about the advantages of the so-named Mediterranean diet. This diet is high in the following food items:

- Soy-based products
- Red grapes, including red wine and grape juice
- Peas and legumes (various kinds of beans)
- Citrus fruits
- Raspberries
- Strawberries
- Blueberries
- Fish
- Aged garlic (over one year)
- Green tea

A nutrient in food known as beta-carotene also helps to slow the growth of cancer cells. This is found in such foods as these:

- Leafy green vegetables
- Broccoli

- Spinach
- Kale
- Romaine lettuce
- Beets
- Carrots
- Swiss chard
- Sweet potatoes
- Yams

Vitamin E and selenium. Much has been written about the value of certain dietary supplements, such as selenium and vitamin E, as products that can reduce the risk of prostate cancer. The suggested daily dosage is usually said to be a 200-microgram pill of selenium and 15 milligrams of vitamin E. However, these are dietary supplements that should be added to the recommended foods listed above. Bear in mind that vitamin E can also be consumed through the regular diet and without the use of supplements.

A scientific study called SELECT, which is intended to more accurately determine the nutritional value of selenium and vitamin E supplements and their effectiveness in preventing or slowing the spread of prostate cancer, began right here in my home city of Cleveland, Ohio, in 2001. The study is directed by Dr. Eric Klein of the Cleveland Clinic Foundation, who is also the head of urologic oncology at that hospital. "Previous studies have hinted that these nutrients may reduce the chance of getting prostate cancer by controlling the cell damage that leads to cancer."[17]

More than four hundred medical centers in the United States, Canada, and Puerto Rico are expected to enroll 32,400 men in the SELECT trial over the next four years. SELECT, which is sponsored by the National Cancer Institute, will span more than twelve years.[18] My friend Michael R. White, who is a former three-term mayor of Cleveland, has enrolled in this study. He did so in large measure because he is now fifty years old, his father has been diagnosed with this disease, and his grandfather died from prostate cancer.[19] Family history places him at risk for developing prostate cancer. (Men interested in participating in this study may call the National Cancer Institute at 1-800-4-CANCER or visit the NCI website at www.cancer.gov.)

Apples. I mentioned earlier that I was in elementary school when I first heard the saying "An apple a day keeps the doctor away." As it turns out, that was good medical advice. Patrick Walsh says, "Better yet, an apple, an orange, a bowl of vegetable soup and maybe some corn on the cob. . . . But simply eating an apple gives your body far more antioxidant and cancer-fighting help than taking mega doses of vitamins."[20]

Bear in mind that diet and lifestyle changes alone are not a guarantee that you will avoid developing prostate cancer. Everything in this chapter must be considered: age, race or ethnicity, environment, and family history. Add to those risk factors the importance of beginning prostate cancer screening with the PSA blood test and the digital rectal exam as early as forty years of age but certainly no later than fifty. However, you can reduce your risk of developing prostate cancer or at least slow the spread of cancer that has already developed by following the dietary suggestions and lifestyle changes that are recommended by the American Cancer Society and by your family physician or your urologist.

Questions to Consider

♦ Do you fit into any of the groups that are at high risk for prostate cancer, based on age, race or ethnicity, environment, or family history?

♦ Has any other member of your family ever been diagnosed with prostate cancer? Have you considered both your father and mother's side of the family?

✠ Do you still consume a high-fat diet that includes large amounts of red meat and dairy products (whole milk, cheeses, whole butter, ice cream, and so on)?

✠ Do you consume a large amount of foods that are high in sugar, such as cookies, candy bars, ice cream, and most soft drinks?

✠ Do you know that lean meats are better for you than processed meats like cold cuts?

✠ Do you know the foods that constitute the so-named Mediterranean diet?

✠ Are you aware of the nutritional and anticancer benefits of tomatoes and other foods that are high in lycopene?

✠ Do you consume five or more servings of fresh fruits and vegetables every day?

✠ Did you know that leafy green vegetables, like collard or turnip greens, broccoli, kale, spinach, or romaine lettuce, can reduce your risk of developing prostate cancer?

✠ Do you practice the old adage that "An apple a day keeps the doctor away"?

✠ Have you made any of the lifestyle changes suggested in this chapter that can help to reduce your risk of developing prostate cancer?

NOTES

1. Joseph E. Oesterling and Mark A. Moyad, *The ABCs of Prostate Cancer: The Book That Could Save Your Life* (Lanham, MD: Madison, 2003), p. 8.

2. American Cancer Society, *Facts on Prostate Cancer and Prostate Cancer Testing, 2002*, p. 3.

3. Oesterling and Moyad, *ABCs of Prostate Cancer*, p. 10.

4. Ibid., p. 12.

5. Ibid., p. 11.

6. Patrick Walsh and Janet Farrar Worthington, *Dr. Patrick Walsh's Guide*

to *Surviving Prostate Cancer* (New York: Warner, 2001), pp. 63–64.

7. Sheldon Marks, *Prostate and Cancer: A Family Guide to Diagnosis, Treatment, and Survival* (Cambridge, MA: Fisher, 1999), p. 21.

8. Ibid., p. 21.

9. Ibid., p. 25.

10. American Cancer Society, *Facts on Prostate Cancer,* p. 3.

11. Walsh and Worthington, *Dr. Patrick Walsh's Guide,* p. 79.

12. Ibid.

13. Marks, *Prostate and Cancer,* p. 28.

14. Walsh and Worthington, *Dr. Patrick Walsh's Guide,* p. 78.

15. Ibid., p. 80.

16. Oesterling and Moyad, *ABCs of Prostate Cancer,* p. 13.

17. Josette Compton, "African American Men Most Susceptible to Prostate Cancer," *The Call and Post,* January 16, 2004, p. A4.

18. Ibid.

19. Ibid.

20. Walsh and Worthington, *Dr. Patrick Walsh's Guide,* p. 97.

7

Realizing We Are Not Alone

"We all need somebody to lean on."
—"Lean on Me," Bill Withers

TODAY I AM A CANCER SURVIVOR LIVING AN ACTIVE LIFE and doing everything I can to encourage other men to pay attention to this area of their health. But the day I was diagnosed with prostate cancer was the loneliest day of my life. Within a matter of a few weeks, my world had been turned upside down. When my prostate cancer was finally confirmed, I had never felt more frightened, confused, and alone.

The "Old Man's Disease"

I had heard about prostate cancer over the years, and I had known several men who had contracted this disease. These men were, on average, in their late sixties and early seventies, and that seemed consistent with what I believed about prostate cancer—that it was a disease for older men. When I was diagnosed, I was fifty-four years old, in otherwise excellent health, and with no physical symptoms of any kind. I had no pain in the groin area or the lower back. I had no difficulty with my bladder, no pain in passing water, and no blood in my urine. All I had was a slightly elevated PSA score, and that is what set in motion a series of events that resulted in my being diagnosed and treated for prostate cancer.

Cancer was a word I had often heard associated with other people, but I never thought I would hear that word associated with me. In my thirty years of pastoral ministry in New York, New Jersey, and now Ohio, I had visited countless people who had contracted one of the many forms of cancer. I had presided at the funerals of innumerable men and women who eventually died from the devastating effects of cancer. I was not at all unfamiliar with the disease, but like most people who contract cancer, I was unprepared to hear that I had developed this disease.

Part of the shock of my diagnosis was not only that I had contracted the disease. Rather, this experience was a rude awakening to the fact that time had not been standing still in my life and that I was now old enough to be a candidate for prostate cancer. I started out in the ministry at the age of twenty-three. I was ordained at the age of twenty-five, and I was called to my first job as the pastor of a congregation at the age of twenty-six. I was always "the young minister" or the "youthful pastor." Even when I came to this large congregation in Cleveland, I was only thirty-eight years old, and I was still thinking of myself as young and youthful.

I should have realized that something had changed when I received in the mail an unsolicited membership application from AARP (the American Association of Retired Persons). Then the Social Security Administration sent me a projection of what my retirement check ("old age pension") would be. Shortly after that, I received an invitation to my thirtieth class reunion from graduate school. Despite all of those indicators, however, my middle-age status did not fully strike home. When I was diagnosed with prostate cancer, a disease even I had known was most prevalent among "older men," I could not believe I was really that old.

Someone to Lean On

My most immediate reaction, after fear and anxiety, was that I needed someone I could turn to and lean on as I made my way through whatever lay ahead for me. In the hours after I had received that phone call from the urologist, I kept asking myself, "What am I going to do?" and "How am I going to make it through this?" I knew that I could lean on my wife. I shared the news with her right away, and she has been a strong source of support and encouragement from the beginning of this process. However, the cancer was not inside her body; it was inside mine. And so there was only so much help and encouragement she could offer. She was unable to answer the questions that raced through my mind about the severity of and treatment for the disease I was now confronting.

I never doubted that my faith in God was strong or that God's presence would undergird me through the process. Nevertheless, I had some questions that burdened me, not just from time to time, but constantly. How advanced was my cancer? What treatment options were available? I had heard about the side effects of prostate cancer treatment; would I face those challenges? Was my life in danger, and if so, how long did I have left to live? Why was this happening to me? Almost from the moment I received my diagnosis, my mind was flooded with questions like these. I prayed about all of these concerns, but it seemed that God was not volunteering much information on this subject. So there I was—shocked by the news, frightened about what the future held for me, and feeling like I was alone, with no one to talk to and no one who really understood what I was feeling.

Then it happened. Men in the church and men in the community who were prostate cancer survivors began approaching me on an almost daily basis with words of support and encouragement. I had no idea how prevalent prostate cancer was in our society until those men began making themselves known to me. "Rev, I've been there, and you'll be all right." "Doc, I'm an eight-year survivor, and it will be all right." "Mac, you just hang in there. I've been where you are going, and if you need me, I'll be right there with you." From the moment I shared the news of my diagnosis with the deacons of our church and later with the congregation, I was overwhelmed by the encouragement that was given to me, not from people who were simply well-wishers, but from men who were prostate cancer survivors.

That was what I needed. I was thinking of myself as a victim of prostate cancer, with nothing to look forward to but a worsening condition and a shortened life span. These men were prostate cancer *survivors* who had been through what I was now facing and were getting on with their lives. They looked healthy and vigorous; they were no longer suffering from any of the side effects; and most of all, they were uniformly optimistic that I would be fine when the treatment was over. I began to realize that prostate cancer is a serious disease that has the potential to kill, but when detected at an early stage, and when met with an appropriate treatment, it can be cured.

These survivors began to share their stories with me—stories about the treatment options they had chosen, about the side effects they had experienced, about the fear that had gripped them when they were first diagnosed. And many of them spoke to me about the normalcy that had returned to their lives in the years since their prostate cancer had been cured. I was no longer alone. Others had been through what was now facing me, and every one of them who made themselves known urged me to call upon them whenever I had any question or concern about what was lying ahead for me.

I can honestly say that throughout my battle with prostate cancer one of the most important resources I had was the awareness of how many other men around me had already fought and won their own battle with the same killer disease. In addition to those who spoke to me in person, telephone calls started coming to my house from men who had either already been treated for this sickness or were going through their treatment at the present time. They had heard my announcement in the sermons I had preached in the weeks leading up to my surgery, and they called me in their capacity as survivors and as former sufferers to pray with me and to assure me that I, too, would soon be a prostate cancer survivor.

The calls did not come only in the days leading up to my surgery; they also came after I had been released from the hospital and was at home recuperating. One day I got a call from a man with whom I had worked over the years in several civic projects. He called to tell me that he had been through the same surgery on the same day at the same hour at another hospital in Cleveland. We swapped stories about how we were feeling and how we were coping with the catheter. We talked about what we were both looking forward to doing in the weeks and months ahead when our recovery was complete.

It seemed that with every passing day I came to realize two important things. First, prostate cancer is prevalent in our society and men need to pay attention to this disease by being screened annually through the digital rectal exam and the PSA blood test. Second, I came to realize that prostate cancer can be cured if it is detected early and treated properly. That knowledge, regularly reinforced by scores of prostate cancer survivors, was exactly what I needed in order to win my battle against this disease.

Telling the Deacons

I broke the news about my elevated PSA score to our board of deacons at their monthly meeting in March. This was before the biopsy had confirmed the presence of cancer in my body, but I wanted to get people praying for me as soon as possible. I claimed the language of James 5:14-15 that says, "Is any among you sick? Let him call for the elders of the church and let them pray over him . . . the prayer of faith shall save the sick." When I shared my news with the elders of our church, they surrounded me, laid hands on me, and began to pray for my healing as well as for my family and my ministry. It was a powerful moment for me, because I had much more experience at praying for others than I had in having others pray for me.

However, as powerful as the prayers were, what moved and encouraged me most were the testimonies that began to be shared from the male deacons in that room who revealed, some of them for the first time, that they, too, had been through prostate cancer. We have a board of deacons made up of thirty-five members, thirty of whom are males. Of those thirty, eight had battled this disease, and five of them had been treated for it within the last year. Those men had opted for different treatments, so I now had available to me men who had recent experience with the radical prostatectomy, radiation therapy, and hormone therapy.

Those men began to share with me the books, pamphlets, Internet sites, and doctors' advice that had been helpful to them when they were going through the process. They continued to call me at home in the evenings and to stop by the house and talk with me about what I was experiencing. They understood the feelings I had. They patiently answered all of my questions, even when I asked them about such things as incontinence and impotence, the two most dreaded potential side effects of prostate cancer treatment.

However, the most important thing they did for me was to assure me—simply by their being alive and active—that people can be diagnosed and treated for this disease and then can get on with their lives. Their living witness, as well as their spoken words and heartfelt prayers, was just what I needed in the days and weeks following my own diagnosis. It was their willingness to share with me about their experiences in so open a manner that caused me to make the commitment, following my own cancer treatment, to devote a considerable part of the rest of my life to doing the same thing for other men. Writing this book is a part of that commitment!

My Clergy Colleagues

Not only did I discover that I was not the only man in my church to have prostate cancer; I quickly discovered that neither was I the only clergyman in Cleveland to have this disease. Dr. Dennis Norris, the executive minister of the Cleveland Baptist Association, and Bishop J. Delano Ellis, presiding bishop of the United Pentecostal Churches of Christ (with headquarters in Cleveland), had both been quite public about their bouts with this disease several years earlier and about the radical prostatectomies they had been through. I called them and spoke with them at length about my condition. The fact that they had been open about their experiences in the past opened the door for me to talk with them about what I could expect in the future.

On the day before I went into the hospital for surgery, Dr. Norris and his wife came to my home to pray with my wife and me. On the day of the surgery, Bishop Ellis met me at the hospital, prayed with me just before I went into the operating room, stayed with my wife throughout the entire procedure, and was the first face I saw when I was being rolled from the recovery room to a regular room in the hospital. I had been the pastor for many people who were facing serious illnesses and major surgery, but now I needed someone to serve in that capacity on my behalf. These two men were there for me and for my family. Once again, I praise God that I was not alone.

Rev. Vincent Miller is a member of my local clergy association, United Pastors in Mission, and a one-year prostate cancer survivor. He, too, had spoken about his battle with this disease during several of our weekly meetings. In the weeks after my diagnosis, I spoke with him at length on several occasions. He had opted for the radiation therapy using seed implants, so I was able to talk with him about the pros and cons of that approach. We see each other at our weekly meetings, and not once since I returned to the group after my surgery have we failed to ask each other how we are doing. Here again, one man's openness about his battle with prostate cancer provided me with someone with whom I could talk and pray about my condition. I was not alone.

After I announced that I had been diagnosed with prostate cancer and was about to have surgery, one of the local community newspapers interviewed me and then ran a story about it. Two other pastors, Rev. Jewel Jones and Rev. David Hunter, who had not heard about my condition until they read about it in that newspaper, called me on the phone to offer their support, and both of them remain in regular contact with me to this day. They both had the same procedure that I underwent, so they were invaluable in helping me deal with the annoyance of the catheter, the impatience, and the cabin fever I experienced during the six weeks of recuperation at home, not to mention my frustration with the slow recovery from the side effects.

It seemed as if every day saw some other man calling me or dropping me a note to tell me that he was also dealing with prostate cancer. I have had great conversations with other prostate cancer survivors while standing in line in the grocery store, the post office, the receiving line at church after the Sunday services, or while waiting to get some popcorn at the movie theater. Dozens of men have also since called me because they have been diagnosed with prostate cancer and they need a shoulder to lean on, an ear to listen while they discuss their fears and anxieties, and some recent experience they can draw upon as they decide how to proceed with their treatment for this disease.

Prostate Cancer as a Ministry Opportunity

I have come to understand that being stricken with prostate cancer served an important purpose in my life. I now think of this experience as God putting me in a position where my ministry could be strengthened, expanded, and perhaps even redefined. As I said in the first chapter of this book, this was an opportunity to model for others, in my congregation and beyond, what it looked like to be "sick and saved." I had told other people to trust in God when they were going through some serious sickness, and now it was my time to practice in my own life what I had been preaching to others. If I did not demonstrate this principle of being sick and saved now, when the entire church and the wider community were aware of my condition, I would have little credibility later on when I tried to encourage other people to "keep the faith" when a serious sickness was confronting them. This was a test I had to pass!

Next, I saw this experience as an opportunity to become an advocate for prostate cancer screening and early detection. I have been a high-profile person in Cleveland for the last fifteen years, regularly appearing in local media as a result of my involvement in issues of civil rights, workers' rights, economic development, HIV/AIDS, public education, and a wide range of political activities, including a campaign for election to the U.S. House of Representatives in 1998 and to the United States Senate in 2000. In the Democratic Party primary for the U.S. Senate, I ran a statewide campaign, I was profiled in every major newspaper in Ohio, and on Election Day I received more than 230,000 votes. That campaign resulted in a level of public visibility that not many other people in Ohio have achieved.

The question was always being raised about what office I might seek next or about how I planned to translate those 230,000 votes into the building blocks for some future campaign. Then I was diagnosed with prostate cancer, and it quickly became apparent what I should do. Here was a chance to take that high public profile and use it to direct attention to the issue of prostate cancer. I believe that many men have contracted and subsequently died from this disease because it has still not received as much public attention and discussion as it deserves.

I must continue to insert this grim statistic: 220,900 men are diagnosed with prostate cancer, and 28,900 men die from this disease every year. Dr. Patrick Walsh of Johns Hopkins University is one of the world's leading experts on the treatment of prostate cancer, and he describes these statistics in even starker terms when he observes that "every three minutes a man is diagnosed with prostate cancer and every sixteen minutes a man dies from this disease."[1] It is for that reason that I have gone to health fairs, done radio interviews, and written this book. I have even looked for ways to work the issue of prostate cancer into as many of my sermons and speeches as possible. I am determined to use every communications outlet available to me to encourage men to be aware of the dangers of, and the treatments for, this potentially deadly disease.

I have also committed myself to talking one-on-one with any man who calls me and says he has been diagnosed with prostate cancer. I know the shock and fear that comes with that diagnosis. I know how anxious I was when I first received that news. Most of all, I know what a comfort and an encouragement it was for me when prostate cancer survivors made themselves available to me. My ministry has literally been redefined by this experience of sickness. I can now be helpful to a group of men and their families in ways that were not possible before I became a cancer survivor. Even people who are battling other forms of cancer desire to speak with a person who has come through a prostate cancer experience. One of the ways I made the move from "Why me?" to "What next?" was to turn my personal experience as a cancer patient into a ministry opportunity as a cancer survivor.

Prostate Cancer Victims

The battle against prostate cancer has been greatly aided by a long list of nationally known celebrities who have been willing to reveal that they have contracted this disease. If any man thinks he is alone in this struggle, all he needs to do is consider the men of national and even international prominence who have been treated for, have died from, or have recently learned that they had contracted prostate cancer. The willingness of these men to release the details about their condition makes it easier to achieve broad, national awareness about prostate cancer detection and treatment.

Dr. Benjamin S. Carson Sr. The news that I had developed prostate cancer coincided with the release of the January 2003 issue of *Ebony* magazine, which reported that the world-famous neurosurgeon Dr. Ben Carson of Johns Hopkins University had recently battled this disease. He was fifty years old when he was diagnosed, so like me, he was at the younger end of the scale so far as developing this disease is concerned. Carson underwent a surgical procedure to remove the cancer from his body.[2]

In the September 2003 issue of *Ebony,* an issue that listed the names and testimonies of numerous, prominent African Americans Carson stated, "Prostate cancer doesn't have to kill anyone. The diseases of the prostate gland are eminently treatable if detected early and treated aggressively. There is no reason that a person diagnosed with these diseases cannot live a long, productive and highly enjoyable life."[3] Hearing that testimony at precisely the time when I was recovering from prostate cancer surgery was a great source of encouragement for me, and it also helped me to make my decision to be an advocate for prostate cancer.

John Kerry. The next nationally known person who went public about his battle with prostate cancer was United States Senator John Kerry from Massachusetts, who was treated for the disease in February 2003. At the time of his treatment he was also among the leading contenders for the nomination of the Democratic Party for the office of president of the United States of America in 2004. Kerry opted for the radical prostatectomy and spent three days in the hospital. However, upon his release from the hospital, he did not take the customary four to six weeks to recover from the surgery. Instead, he resumed his campaign schedule and soon clinched the Democratic nomination.

I took great interest in his case, because it was a reminder that a man can have cancer surgery and then resume an active lifestyle. I watched Kerry's campaign closely while I was going through my own cancer treatment and while I was working on this book. I was interested in his ability to recover from prostate surgery and face the rigors of a presidential campaign.

My urologist and much of the literature about prostate cancer suggest that a person can resume an active schedule even before the catheter is removed, switching between the large Foley bag that is used at night to capture urine and the smaller leg bag that serves the same purpose but fits around the thigh and allows a person to move more freely during the day. Once the catheter is removed (usually two or three weeks after the surgery), some people actually try to return to work, with the only restriction being that they not lift anything that weighs more than ten or twenty pounds.[4] That is apparently what John Kerry decided to do.

Robert DeNiro. On October 20, 2003, it was announced that the actor Robert DeNiro had been diagnosed with this disease at the age of sixty. Given his immense popularity and prominence as a two-time Academy Award–winning movie star with a film career that had stretched over forty years, the issue of prostate cancer was once again front page news all across the country. The specific cancer treatment that he opted for was not released. However, the fact that a man who has played as many tough-guy film roles as Robert DeNiro was now fighting a real-life battle with a life-threatening disease undoubtedly captured the attention of men across the country and around the world. If it could happen to Robert DeNiro, it could happen to any middle-aged man.

Colin Powell. On December 15, 2003, it was revealed that Colin Powell, the secretary of state of the United States, a former chairman of the Joint Chiefs of Staff of the U.S. military, and a retired four-star general of the United States Army, had been battling prostate cancer for some time. The announcement coincided with his undergoing a radical prostatectomy at the age of sixty-six. Here again, the fact that Powell had been a national leader in Washington, D.C., for over a decade made his announcement about prostate cancer all the more significant. He took off a few weeks after his surgery to recover, but by early January 2004, he was back to the grueling schedule associated with being the chief diplomatic spokesperson for the United States government. He was also being interviewed on various TV programs, and always the issue of his being a prostate cancer survivor was a part of the discussion.

Here is a sample listing of other prominent men who have been diagnosed with prostate cancer, many of whom survive to this day. (*Asterisk indicates now deceased.)

Government officials

- Marion Barry, former mayor of Washington, D.C.
- Robert Dole, former U.S. senator from Kansas
- Rudolph Giuliani, former mayor of New York City
- Jesse Helms, former U.S. senator from North Carolina
- Richard Shelby, current U.S. senator from Alabama
- John Paul Stevens, associate justice of the United States Supreme Court
- Ted Stevens, current U.S. senator from Alaska
- Louis Sullivan, former secretary of health and human services
- Andrew Young, former mayor of Atlanta and U.S. ambassador to the U.N.

Entertainers

- Don Ameche, actor*
- Harry Belafonte, actor, singer, and humanitarian
- Bill Bixby, actor (*The Incredible Hulk* TV series)*
- Robert Goulet, singer and actor
- Jerry Lewis, comedian and actor
- Sidney Poitier, actor and director
- Telly Savalas, actor (*Kojak* TV series)*
- Frank Zappa, singer and musician*

Athletes and coaches

- Dusty Baker, manager of the Chicago Cubs (baseball)
- Len Dawson, former quarterback for the Kansas City Chiefs (football)
- Marv Levy, former head coach of the Buffalo Bills (football)
- Stan Musial, Hall of Fame player with the St. Louis Cardinals (baseball)
- Arnold Palmer, golfer and golf course designer
- Richard Petty, champion race car driver in the Winston Cup circuit

- Bobby Riggs, player of historic match against Billie Jean King (tennis)
- Frank Robinson, Hall of Fame player with the Baltimore Orioles (baseball)
- Joe Torre, manager of the New York Yankees (baseball)

Other prominent men
- Les Brown, motivational speaker
- Stokely Carmichael, civil rights activist who coined the term "Black Power"*
- Louis Farrakhan, leader of the Nation of Islam
- Nelson Mandela, former president of South Africa
- Robert Novak, syndicated columnist and host of CNN's *Crossfire*
- Pat Robertson, clergyman and founder of The 700 Club
- H. Norman Schwarzkopf, United States Army General, retired
- Desmond Tutu, bishop and antiapartheid activist in South Africa
- Cornel West, scholar and writer now teaching at Princeton University

As you consider this list of high-profile men who have been willing to go public about their battles with prostate cancer, remember that they are but the tip of the iceberg when it comes to the men affected by this disease. And as my friend and colleague Otis Moss Jr. observed in a recent meeting about prostate cancer in the black community, the impact extends beyond the individual man who has the disease, for it touches his family, his coworkers, and any other individuals or groups who may be influenced by his illness or death. Prostate cancer is a serious health concern for millions of men. Remember the words of Patrick Walsh, who not only reminds us of the 220,900 men who are diagnosed with this disease each year and the 28,900 men who die as a result of prostate cancer. He puts it even more graphically when he says, "Every three minutes another case of prostate cancer is diagnosed and every sixteen minutes a man dies from this disease."[5]

The all-important difference between men being diagnosed with prostate cancer (every three minutes) and men dying from prostate cancer (every sixteen minutes) is early detection and prompt treatment that is appropriate for their age, their overall health, and the grade and stage of the cancer that has been detected. Almost all of the men listed above won their battle with prostate cancer as a result of these two actions. As Ben Carson stated, "Prostate cancer can be treated if it is detected early and treated aggressively."[6] In fact, prostate cancer can be completely cured and men can expect to live a normal life span after they have completed their preferred treatment. Even when the cancer has advanced beyond the stage where a cure is possible, men may live for many years after their diagnosis with treatments that slow the growth and spread of the cancer.

You are not alone in your battle with prostate cancer. There are survivors in every church, in every neighborhood, and in every sector of society. If you are willing to speak up about the cancer you are fighting, someone who has already been through the process will find you and encourage you and assure you that with early detection, prompt and appropriate treatment, and a strong faith in God, you can win this fight. Once you have done so, do not hesitate to pass on to other men the same information and encouragement that was given to you. Prostate cancer survivors constitute a unique fraternity; nobody wants to join the group, but once you are in, you quickly discover that we bear one another's burdens.

Strengthening Your Brothers

In Luke 22:31-32, Jesus tells Simon Peter, "Satan has asked to sift you as wheat. But I have prayed for you, Simon, that your faith may not fail. And when you have turned back, strengthen your brothers" (NIV). These words were spoken on the night when Peter would deny knowing Jesus on three separate occasions. Jesus knew what was going to happen; he knew about Peter's denials, about Judas's betrayal, and about all the other disciples fleeing and leaving him to face his torturous death alone. In the moments before that series of events began to unfold, Jesus was issuing a challenge to Peter: "When all of this is over and you have recovered your faith, be a source of strength for the other disciples."

I want to issue a similar challenge to every prostate cancer survivor. When you have come through, strengthen your brothers. Being diagnosed with cancer is much like being sifted. Every aspect of your character—your faith in God, your will to live, your concern for those who are affected by your condition—is put to the test. Every man who survives prostate cancer has an opportunity to become a source of strength for another man who is about to begin his journey into the valley of the shadow of death.

Until recently, men did not discuss the fact that they had contracted prostate cancer. Even worse than that, many men who were aware of the dangers posed by this disease did not take advantage of the screenings that were made available to them even when they were conveniently offered in a neighborhood center, in a doctor's office, or in the basement of their local church. That silence, coupled with a reluctance to be screened, has undoubtedly resulted in the deaths of thousands of men. It is long past the time to break the silence and to seize upon medical knowledge that can save lives.

The most important voices in the battle against prostate cancer are not the voices of urologists or other physicians; the most important voices are of the survivors. The voices of prostate cancer survivors *must* be heard, and the stories about their survival *must* be told! Our willingness to speak about our personal experience with detection, diagnosis, treatment, and survival will motivate other men to pay closer attention to this aspect of their health. If we are willing to speak about what has happened in our lives, we might be able to help save the lives of others. At that moment we cease to be cancer victims and start becoming cancer awareness advocates. There are few things we will ever do in life that will be of greater importance or that will result in a greater reward.

NOTES

1. Patrick Walsh and Janet Farrar Worthington, *Dr. Patrick Walsh's Guide to Surviving Prostate Cancer* (New York: Warner, 2001), p. 42.
2. Kevin Chappell, "Dr. Ben Carson: Top Surgeon's Life-and-Death Struggle with Prostate Cancer," *Ebony*, January 2003, p. 38.
3. Kevin Chappell, "Life after Prostate Cancer: NMA and Top Leaders Launch Campaign against Leading Killer of Black Men," *Ebony*, September 2003, p. 190.
4. Walsh and Worthington, *Dr. Patrick Walsh's Guide,* pp. 229–36.
5. Ibid., p. 42.
6. Chappell, "Life after Prostate Cancer," p. 190.

8

Walking by Faith

"Your faith has healed you.
Go in peace and be freed from your suffering."
—Mark 5:34, NIV

ONE OF THE STRONGEST AND CLEAREST MESSAGES ANY-
where in the Bible is found within the eleventh chapter of
Hebrews when the writer declares, "Without faith it is impossible to please God" (verse 6, NIV). The writer seems to be telling
us that whatever else we may say or think or do as a Christian,
our relationship with God ultimately depends upon our ability to
take actions that are anchored not in facts but in faith. All the
way through the Bible we are confronted with people who
embraced certain ideas and who embarked upon a certain course
of action, equipped with nothing more than faith in God. Let me
say at the outset of this chapter, therefore, that what is most
important in our development as Christians is not that we join
the church and become active in the various auxiliaries and ministries; what is most important is that we are steadily increasing
our capacity to live and act in faith.

Biblical Examples

The people listed in Hebrews 11 mastered their fears, set aside
their doubts, overcame the objections of others, and then stepped
out in faith. When Noah obeyed God and began the construction

of an ark, a boat meant to carry heavy cargo in deep water, he was living in the desert (Genesis 6–8). Nevertheless, he did what God asked of him as an act of faith.

When Abraham left the security of his home and at age seventy-five began a difficult journey to an unknown destination in Genesis 12, he did not tell God that he was too old or that the request was unreasonable, though both of those objections were true. Abraham obeyed God as an act of faith.

When God called to Moses out of a burning bush in Exodus 3 and told him to return to Egypt and deliver the Hebrew people from their 430 years of slavery to the pharaohs, Moses did not try to explain to God that he was a fugitive from Egyptian justice. He did not try to remind God that the reason he was on Mount Sinai is because he had been hiding there for forty years after he had killed an Egyptian who had been beating a Hebrew slave. Moses did not trouble God with that factual detail; he just obeyed God and returned to Egypt to begin that perilous task as a simple act of faith.

The same can be said for Joshua in Joshua 6, when he conquered the city of Jericho not with swords and spears but by the blowing of trumpets after the people had marched around the walls seven times.

In every case I have listed, the people involved were severely lacking in facts, but they were supremely equipped with faith. Hebrews 11:6 must become the heart and soul of every Christian's daily walk: "Without faith it is impossible to please God."

The examples of walking by faith continue into the New Testament. When the twelve disciples of Jesus left the work they had been doing and became his followers, knowing that birds had nests and foxes had holes but the Son of Man had no place to lay his head (Luke 9:58), theirs was an act of faith. When the Roman soldier standing at the foot of the cross looked up at the dead body of Jesus and then declared, "Surely he was the Son of God!"

(Matthew 27:54, NIV), that shift from executioner to evangelist was a marvelous act of faith. When Saul of Tarsus, who had been an enemy of the church of Jesus Christ, experienced a change of both his name and mission and became the primary ambassador of Jesus Christ to the ancient world in Acts 9, his transformation was an act of faith. In fact, at the end of his life, it was Paul who said, "I have fought the good fight, I have finished the race, I have kept the faith" (2 Timothy 4:7, NIV).

From one end of the Bible to the other—from the announcement that everything that exists was made by the hand of a sovereign God to the announcement that Christ will reign supreme over the whole of creation at the end of time—we are confronted with claims that can be embraced only by faith. On what basis do I declare that Jesus was born from the womb of a virgin girl? It is an act of faith. On what basis do I suggest that Jesus, who was certainly killed and buried following his crucifixion, was raised from the dead three days later? That is a statement of faith. And on what basis do I say that the day is surely coming when, at the name of Jesus, every knee will bow and every tongue will confess that Jesus Christ is Lord to the glory of God the Father? That, too, is an awesome act of faith.

Facing the Diagnosis with Faith

How strong is your faith in the teachings of the Bible and in the promises of God? Faith, says Hebrews 11:1, is "being sure of what we hope for and certain of what we do not see" (NIV). Faith is not waiting until we know all the facts beyond a shadow of a doubt and then acting. Faith is acting even when we do not know, because we trust the God who made the promise. Faith is not guessing or wagering or trusting in probable cause or operating on the basis of whether the odds are for us or against us. Faith is hearing what God is telling us to do, then doing it, whether it seems to make sense at the time or not. Faith is not taking out an insurance policy prior to engaging in a certain course of action so that we are protected if things should go wrong. Faith is risking what is most precious to us, but doing it because we believe that God is with us and will see us through.

How strong is your faith in God? What is the last thing you did solely as an act of faith? Before you answer that question, let me remind you of the faith shown by some people whose names and actions are most likely familiar to you. When Harriet Tubman made her nineteen journeys into slaveholding regions of the United States to deliver over three hundred people from slavery in the South to freedom in Canada, what was her motivation and her inspiration? It was her faith in God. When Mary McLeod Bethune began a university for black people in Daytona Beach, Florida, in 1904, what did she have with which to begin? Her answer was "Faith and a dollar and a half." When Rosa Parks sat down on a bus in Montgomery in 1955, when Martin Luther King Jr. stood up for freedom in Birmingham in 1963, or when John Lewis led a group of marchers into the teeth of the Alabama State Patrol on the Edmund Pettus Bridge in Selma in 1965, what was it that enabled each of them to do what they did? The answer is the same in every case: it was their faith.

Faith is our willingness to embrace an idea that others are rejecting, because we believe that idea to be true. Faith is our willingness to engage in an action from which others turn away for one reason or another, because we believe that action to be just or moral or godly. Most of all, faith is our willingness to face a risk or endure a loss or go for some period of time without knowing how things are going to turn out in the end, because we believe that what we are involved in is the will of God for our lives at that point in time.

Walking by Faith, Not by Sight

Winning the battle against prostate cancer is as much an act of faith as it is a feat of medicine. When we are first diagnosed with cancer, we do not know how things are going to be resolved. We do not know if the cancer has already spread so far that most treatment options are futile so far as being cured is concerned. When we opt for a particular treatment approach, we are not sure whether all the cancer has been removed or whether further radiation and chemotherapy will be needed to finish the job. We do not know how long the side effects will last or even if they will go away at all.

So many unknowns arise following a cancer diagnosis that it can leave some men and their families overwhelmed with fear and frustration. *Am I going to live? How long do I have to live? Will I have to wear padded underwear for an indefinite period of time to safeguard against urine leaks? Will I ever again be able to share sexual intimacy with my wife?* Even though our doctors assure us that most of our anxieties are unfounded, we all know of men diagnosed with prostate cancer for whom all of these concerns are now daily facts of life. It is precisely at this point when we do not and cannot fully know how things are ultimately going to work out that faith becomes an invaluable resource.

I remember the most frightening time in my battle with prostate cancer. It was not the day I was diagnosed, though that day was frightening enough. It was not even the day of the surgery, because that was at least a step on the road to my treatment and eventual healing. The most frightening time—the time when I was most unnerved by my cancerous condition—was in the two months that followed my biopsy.

My surgeon told me that it took that long for the tissue in and around the prostate to heal after the samples had been taken. The surgery could not be performed until those two months had elapsed. It would have been easy for me to have spent every minute of every day for those two months thinking about nothing but the fact that I had cancer. The only way I was able to endure those two months of waiting and wondering was to draw upon my faith in God. I had to practice what I had been preaching to others. I had to lay claim to the promise of Hebrews 11:1: "Faith is being sure of what we hope for and certain of what we do not see."

God's Faithfulness

I ask you the same question as before. How strong is your faith in God? What is the last thing you did in your life as an expression and an extension of your faith in God? If you are fighting your own battle with prostate cancer (or any other life-threatening disease or debilitating illness), I want to invite you to step out on faith and embrace whatever challenge God is setting before you. You have faced other challenges and crises in the past, and somehow God has brought you through all of them. Now is the time to believe without a doubt that God can bring you through this crisis as well. It is time to walk by faith and not by sight (2 Corinthians 5:7). You've done it before.

God's faithfulness through career moves. There may have been a time when God called you to leave the comfort and security of a steady job and begin a new venture that had been racing through your mind. You acted on faith then, even though you could not know how things were going to work out. Was there a time when you felt God directing you to move from one region of the country to another, but some of your family and closest friends were cautioning against it? Despite their concerns, were you persuaded that the Lord was moving in your life? You relied upon your faith in that situation and found once again that God was reliable.

God's faithfulness with marriage. Marriage, perhaps more than any other human institution, involves a capacity for faith. My wife and I were engaged to be married within three weeks of the day we met, and we were married after knowing each other for less than four months. Almost everybody who knew us, including the man who introduced us on a blind date, told us that it was a mistake for us to get married so quickly. But we knew what we had been looking for in a spouse, and we recognized it in each other. Was there a possibility of things not working out? Of course, but we were willing to act in faith and allow God to lead us down a path that others around us could not or would not see. That was twenty-nine years ago, and there is one thing of which I am convinced: there is little worth having in this life that does not come to us as a result of some major or minor act of faith. "Without faith it is impossible to please God."

God's faithfulness in sickness. The necessity of faith applies not only to our career and marriage decisions but also to our battle with prostate cancer. We do not know precisely what the outcome will be. We cannot be sure, based upon the treatment we select, that the cancer will be eliminated. However, not knowing the facts is no justification for not acting in faith. We must act swiftly and prudently on two fronts: medical and spiritual. We must turn to expert surgeons and time-tested medical procedures on the one hand, and on the other hand we must turn to him who made the blind to see, the lame to walk, and the dead to rise again.

I surrounded myself with as much information as possible so that I could better understand the sickness that had entered my body. But at the same time, I also felt surrounded with the prayers of many people who were encouraging me to believe that God was going to work things out in my life. Now is the time to lay claim to the promise of James 5:16, which says, "The prayer of a righteous man is powerful and effective" (NIV). That was true in my life, and I commend a similar faith to you.

During those two months when I began to dwell on the dangers that awaited me, I had to remind myself of the God who had promised never to leave me alone. On the day of the surgery, when I knew that I would be under anesthesia and not aware of what was happening in that operating room, I had to remind myself that the God I serve neither slumbers nor sleeps (Psalm 121:3-4). In the six weeks of my recuperation (two of them while still wearing a Foley bag), I was encouraged by my assurance that God would put the broken pieces of my life together again. Yes, I had cancer, but I also had faith in God. Today I am cancer free, and it has been my faith in God that has sustained me during this battle with prostate cancer.

This brings me to another point I want to make about faith, and that is the awareness that at various times in your life you will be asked to exercise faith in one of several ways.

Faith's Forms

Faith comes in many forms. We can have faith in ourselves, faith in others (especially medical professionals), and most of all faith in God.

Faith in ourselves. Sometimes your faith must be in yourself and in your God-given abilities. In 1947, when Jackie Robinson and then Larry Doby integrated major league baseball, each of them did so believing that if he were given the opportunity to perform at that level, he could play baseball as well as anybody else who showed up on the field. These men believed that they had God-given talent and ability and they were confident that they could get the job done. Call it self-confidence or self-assurance or any other term or phrase you prefer, but unless you have faith in yourself and in your own abilities, you will not run many risks or take many chances or achieve any great successes in your life.

There is no sin attached to being self-confident or self-assured. There is nothing wrong with having faith in yourself and in your own abilities. Of course, the arrogance that causes some people to look down on others and judge others to be inferior to them is a vile and ugly sin. But when somebody says that God has equipped him or her to do this job or that task, and to do it as well as anybody else in this world, that is not arrogance as much as it is a positive attitude about oneself. I urge you to possess faith in yourself and in your own God-given talents and abilities.

Faith in others. Sometimes faith takes the form of placing trust in others who are around us. When I was in Huntsville, Alabama, for a revival, the host pastor took me to visit the NASA Space and Rocket Center located in that city. I remember standing in front of a replica of the capsule in which John Glenn orbited the earth back in 1962. You cannot imagine how small and tight was the space in which Glenn had to sit for several hours as that capsule first pushed outside of earth's atmosphere, then was sent into a series or orbits around the earth, and finally was brought back to earth for a crash-landing in the ocean. It seems unimaginable that such a thing could be done.

It is certain, however, that John Glenn was not depending upon his own skill as a pilot when he climbed into that rocket. He was placing his life in the hands of others who played the major part in that process. He was demonstrating faith in the people who designed and built the rocket and the capsule. He was putting his faith in the engineers who charted the course he was to follow. He was showing faith in the training he had received from NASA. He was not going through that ordeal by himself; he was putting his faith in the others who were involved with him in that flight around the earth.

Sooner or later, we must all do the same and put our faith in other people and the skills and talents God has given to them. When I get on an airplane, it is an act of faith in the talents of the people who built the plane and the people who are flying it at thirty-five thousand feet in the air. When we order food in a restaurant, we are eating something that we did not grow, did not clean, and did not cook. We are showing enormous faith in the farmers who did grow it and in the cooks and waiters who prepare it and set it before us to eat.

When I went into my surgery on July 31, 2003, I was not planning on operating on myself. I took no crash courses in urology or oncology. I did not try to master the use of a surgeon's scalpel. Instead, I put my faith in the doctors, nurses, medicines, and technologies that God has allowed to exist for our betterment. I put my faith in people who had spent years mastering a science and perfecting skills so that they were ready, willing, and able to attend to my cancerous condition.

My surgeon came highly recommended by my primary physician. The hospital is one of the best in the world, so far as treating cancer is concerned. And there were three nurses, two from my congregation and one who belonged to another church, who agreed to remain with me around the clock while I was in the hospital. I thank God for all of those resources of help and healing, because they were able to do for me what I could not do for myself.

Sometimes we must be ready and willing to show faith in ourselves, and sometimes we must be willing to show just as much faith in others.

Faith in God. The ultimate acts of faith come in those moments when we know that neither we nor anyone else around us is able to do what needs to be done. There are times when the doctors have done all they can do and medicine has offered all that it is capable of providing. In hours like that we turn to God, and these ultimate acts of faith are always preceded by words like those of the hymn that says, "Father, I stretch my hands to thee, No other help I know."

The woman in Mark 5:25 who was still afflicted with a flow of blood after seeing many doctors over a twelve-year period of time had no place to turn but to Jesus. "Father, I stretch my hands to thee." The man in John 5:5 who had been lying as a cripple for thirty-eight years because he could not get himself into the healing waters of the nearby Pool of Bethsaida had no place to turn except to Jesus. "Father, I stretch my hands to thee." Blind Bartimaeus in Mark 10:46 heard that Jesus was going to pass by the place where he was standing, so he began to call out the words "Have mercy on me." The people told him to be quiet, but Bartimaeus was tired of living in the blindness that had limited his life from the day he was born. Bartimaeus had no place to turn except to Jesus. "Father, I stretch my hands to thee."

When Jesus himself was nailed to the cross on Calvary after the "Hosanna" crowd had changed its tune to "Crucify him," and after Peter had denied him and Judas had betrayed him and all the others had deserted him, he had no place to turn but to God. So he cried out, "Father, into thy hands I commend my spirit" (Luke 23:46, KJV). Even Jesus said, "Father, I stretch my hands to thee."

Sooner or later, in the life of every Christian there comes a time when faith in ourselves and when faith in one another will not be sufficient. That is when we will need to place all of our faith and trust and hope in God.

When that day comes in your life, when your battle with cancer begins in earnest, do not worry, because the God we serve is more than faithful. When we are facing a sickness, no matter how serious it may be, the God we serve is more than faithful. The same God who provided a ram in the bush for Abraham will be faithful in our lives. The same God who provided manna from heaven and water from a rock for Israel in the days of Moses will be faithful in our lives. The same God who preserved Daniel in the lions' den, the three Hebrew boys in the fiery furnace, and Paul and Silas in the Philippian jail will be with us no matter what dangers may come our way.

I invite you to look at and learn from the men and women who are listed in Hebrews 11. They were faithful in their generation, no matter what was set before them. Those of us who have battled with a cancer diagnosis must seek to exhibit a similar faith in God. Let the words of Hebrews 12:1 become your words of hope as you imagine that those who were faithful to God in an earlier generation are now looking down from heaven and are observing us we carry on the work that they began: "Since we are surrounded by such a great cloud of witnesses, let us throw off everything that hinders and the sin that so easily entangles, and let us run with perseverance the race marked out for us" (NIV).

9

Resting in God

For I am persuaded, that neither death,
nor life, nor angels, nor principalities, nor powers,
nor things present, nor things to come,
Nor height, nor depth, nor any other creature,
shall be able to separate us from the love of God,
which is in Christ Jesus our Lord.
—Romans 8:38-39, KJV

I BEGAN WRITING THIS FINAL CHAPTER EXACTLY ONE YEAR to the day after my elevated PSA level of 5.2 was detected and my personal battle with prostate cancer began. I am, of course, a physically healthier person now than I was one year ago. I am cancer free, with an undetectable PSA score. I have greatly altered my diet away from the high-fat foods I overindulged in for most of my life. I have also increased my physical exercise by walking one mile per day. However, it is not the change in my physical health that is most important to me. I earnestly believe that my spiritual life has grown stronger and deeper as a result of this battle with prostate cancer.

My faith in God was tested when this process began in January of 2003. Today, one year later, I can declare without hesitation that the God in whom I placed my trust has proved to be faithful. I placed my hands in God's hand when the battle with cancer began, and God has brought me safely through.

God's Unchanging Hand

I remember one of my professors at Union Seminary in New York City telling us a story about the days when he would go for long walks with his young son. Most of the time the son would resist holding his father's hand. He preferred to walk ahead of his father and explore the world around him. One day, however, they came upon a stretch of the road where the branches of the trees hung over the sidewalk and created a corridor of darkness on an otherwise sunny day. When the young boy reached that spot during their walk, he suddenly stopped and waited for his father to catch up to him. Then he reached up for his father's hand and the two of them walked through that darkened area together.

The young boy enjoyed walking alone when everything around him was bright and clear. He felt secure in being on his own so long as he could see what stretched out before him. But when the road ahead became dark and frightening, he did not want to make that part of the journey alone. He wanted to have his father walking by his side. He wanted to have his father hold his hand while they walked through the darkness together.

Many of us know from personal experience just how that young boy felt. One of the most unsettling feelings we can experience comes in those moments when we feel ourselves left alone in the face of some danger or some uncertain and unpleasant circumstance. The trials and tribulations of this life seem all the more painful and frightening when it appears that we must face those approaching problems all by ourselves. We long for a hand that we can hold or, better yet, a hand that can hold us as we make our way through sickness or suffering or setbacks of one kind or another.

In 1995 I was invited to go with a man named Andrew Sternberg to the fiftieth anniversary of his liberation from a Nazi concentration camp nestled in a valley outside Vienna, Austria. The Nazis had forced those Jewish prisoners to dig caves into the mountain where German airplanes could be repaired out of the view of Allied spy planes. The concentration camp was so shrouded by trees, and the nearby mountain peaks were so tall, that the camp could not be seen from the air. Andrew Sternberg told me that what scared him the most was not the horror that took place every day in that death camp. What bothered him the most was that he and his fellow inmates were cut off from the outside world. No one knew where they were. It seemed to them that there was no way anyone could come to their aid. They had the sense that they were alone in the face of one of the worst evils in the history of the world.

It is true that the sense of being left alone in the face of danger is unsettling, but during my battle with prostate cancer, I came to understand more clearly and more personally something I had only talked about in the past. I came to understand that when you are a child of God, and when you place your hand in God's hand, there is no place on earth where you are left to face things alone. The promise of God is that nothing can separate us from divine love. Nothing can separate us from the divine presence. Nothing can separate us from divine power. When you decide to walk with God and put your faith in the Son, Jesus Christ, you will never walk alone. And when you know that you are in the presence of God, the future does not seem as frightening, because you have someone standing by your side.

A beautiful Christian hymn captures the essence of what I am describing. It says, "Trust in him who will not leave you, Whatsoever years may bring, If by earthly friends forsaken Still more closely to him cling."[1]

Absent from the Church, Present with the Lord

Beginning on July 31, 2003, I went through a series of things that I know I could not have handled by myself. Not only that, but in the succeeding months things have worked out in ways that I could never have accomplished by myself. My wife and son sat with me in a room where I waited for nearly three hours for my surgery to begin. But at 2:55 p.m. on July 31, I was taken to a place where they could not go. The man who drove us to the hospital and the pastoral colleague who met me at the hospital that morning sat in the waiting room until the surgery was over. But for three hours I was unable to hold their hands or see their faces or hear their voices.

What I could have discovered only in that moment was that even though the people who came with me to the hospital were not with me, still I was not alone. Of course there were doctors and nurses in that operating room, but theirs is not the presence I have in mind. There was a Great Physician in that room with me. There was the presence of him who made blind eyes see, who made lame men walk, and who made dead men live again.

I had the calm assurance on that day that God had showed up at University Hospital in Cleveland and told the devil that he could not have my life. After the surgery, I spent four days in the hospital and then six weeks at home recuperating. The best way I can describe that period of time is to say that I was absent from the church building but I was present with the Lord.

I believe that God guided every step of that operation. I believe that God kept the cancer from spreading to other parts of my body. I believe that God has healed me and restored me and kept me alive in the face of a disease that had the power to kill me, because God wanted me to return to my ministry with a new witness and a new testimony. God allowed me to return to the church and tell somebody who may be feeling discouraged, "God is with you." And when God is with you, there is no problem or pressure on earth that the two of you cannot handle together.

That is why Paul goes to such lengths in Romans 8 when he lists things that may come into our lives but that will not be able to separate us from the love of God.

No Separation from God

Paul asks, "Who shall separate us from the love of Christ?" (Romans 8:35, NIV). Then he begins to wonder out loud. What about tribulation? Or distress? Or persecution? Or famine? Or nakedness? Or peril? Or the sword? These are some of the things that can intrude upon our lives and leave us wondering if we have anywhere to turn and anyone to turn to for strength or support.

Sometimes it seems that we have done everything God has demanded of us, and yet people are attacking us for no good reason. That is persecution.

Sometimes our resources have run out—our money is gone and our bills are due and we do not know how we are going to make ends meet. That is famine.

Sometimes personal problems keep us up all night pacing the floor and wondering what the end is going to be. That is tribulation and distress.

Sometimes we discover that everything that made our lives comfortable and pleasant has been stripped away. Our health can be broken; our job can be terminated; our relationships can be strained or broken; our world seems empty and barren. That is nakedness.

Sometimes we find ourselves in physical danger, with someone threatening our very lives. The soldiers in Iraq, the victims of September 11, 2001, and all the victims of violence and homicide that we hear about every day are reminders that our lives often face peril and the sword.

I remind you once again that tomorrow is not promised. The world is a dangerous and uncertain place. There is no guarantee that you or I will see next week, much less next year. So the question looms before us, how we can we live with any degree of optimism and enthusiasm in a world where so much can come at us so fast? Paul has the answer to that question. He says, "For I am persuaded . . ."

I like that phrase "I am persuaded." Paul is not telling us what he thinks or what he hopes or even what he has heard from the experiences of others. Paul is telling us what he knows from *his own* personal experience. "Neither death, nor life, nor angels, nor principalities, nor powers, nor things present, nor things to come, nor height, nor depth, nor any other creature, shall be able to separate us from the love of God, which is in Christ Jesus our Lord" (KJV).

Love in Many Forms

The love of God can be revealed in our lives in many forms, and during my battle with prostate cancer, I have experienced many of them.

Sometimes (perhaps more often than we imagine) the love of God is present in the form of the people of God who come to our aid. Have you ever been sick or frightened and you did not know which way to turn, and then a friend or neighbor or church member showed up at your door—and suddenly you were no longer alone? Sometimes God shows up in the form of the people God places around us.

I needed to thank hundreds of people in my own congregation and throughout the Greater Cleveland community for their willingness to be the instruments through whom the love of God was displayed toward me and my family. For example, two nurses in my congregation, Sherdina Williams and Sandra Brooks, took turns with twelve-hour shifts so that at no point was I ever left alone in the hospital.

For six weeks my wife never had to cook a meal, because day after day members of our church and friends in the community brought meals to our house, and they always brought enough for two or three days. Those precious people were another form in which the love of God was flowing into our home.

I received so many cards, fruit baskets, gift certificates, floral arrangements, phone calls, and visits to the house that once again I never felt that I was going through this cancer experience alone. I was absent from the church building, but praise God I was present with the Lord in the form of all the people who prayed for me and showed their love in tangible ways.

Many people agreed to do the shopping for us, bringing in the things we needed so that my wife, Peggy, could concentrate on being the best nurse a man could ever have. She set up a hospital bed for me in a room on the first floor of our home with every comfort and convenience I would need, especially for the first two weeks when I could not climb any stairs. Of course, my son Aaron had to make sure that the angle from the bed to the TV was just right, so he climbed into the bed ahead of me and tested it from every lying and sitting position.

Peggy slept on a sofa every night right beside me. She drove me where I had to go and she fussed at me when she thought that I was doing something I should not be doing. She took seriously the marriage vow that says "in sickness and in health." We have been married since 1975, but during my six weeks of recuperation, she was called upon to display a level of commitment that I had never physically needed before, and she rose to the challenge, allowing the love of God to flow into my life through her.

God showed up at my church, Antioch, for six weeks in a row in the form of the visiting and staff ministers who preached during my absence. The first preacher to fill in for me during my recuperation was also the first preacher with whom I spoke and prayed after I received my cancer diagnosis, Rev. Dr. Otis Moss Jr. I am truly honored that he wrote a foreword for this book.

Every Sunday after church, somebody from Antioch would come by our house and tell us what a wonderful job the preacher had done that day. They would give us a blow-by-blow description of the sermon and of how warmly the preacher was received by the congregation. After a while, I got tired of hearing about how well the service was going without me! The news from Antioch was so good that Peggy and I said to ourselves that maybe we would not go back at all since they seemed to be doing so well without us.

Of course, I was actually chomping at the bit to get back to work, especially to get back to the pulpit. That was the first time in my thirty-year ministry, dating back to my ordination at Abyssinian Baptist Church of New York City in 1973, that I had gone six weeks without preaching. I did not mind having the time away from church administration—that was a blessing. But as those six Sunday mornings came and went, I felt like something essential to my life and identity had been taken away when I was not standing up to preach the gospel message. It does not seem to matter how sick a preacher may be; when Sunday morning rolls around, a preacher wants to preach!

I could not preach for six weeks, but it was a great relief to me to know that the church was in good hands while I was away. It was a joy to know that the congregation was being well fed on Sundays and that the church was being well managed during the week by our marvelous office staff. When you have friends and coworkers who agree to take the burden off your shoulders so that you can concentrate on your surgery and convalescence, that is nothing less than the love of God keeping you from feeling that you are going through something alone.

I Am Persuaded

There is just one more reflection that I want and need to share in this book about battling prostate cancer. I now believe that preachers are made stronger in their proclamation of the gospel when they have to go through something serious themselves. They are better prepared to preach the gospel with all of the power and insight that the task demands—or to hear in the gospel story all of the power and promise it extends to those who believe its message—when they have faced sickness or suffering in their own lives. We preachers can certainly affirm what the Bible says when we preach, and we can comment on what God has done in the lives of others. But that kind of faith and that kind of preaching are largely intellectual and academic, and they have limited power to reach, encourage, and inspire other people who are going through some difficult moments in their lives. Sooner or later we preachers need for life to leave a few scars on our own bodies, a few tear stains on our own cheeks, and some deep concerns about our own continued mortal existence before we have fully earned the right to say, "The Lord will make a way somehow."

The same is true for those who sit in church pews week after week. People need to know what it is like to worry all night about their own health and ponder the possibility of their own death before they fully understand what David meant when he said out of his own experience, "Yea, though I walk through the valley of the shadow of death, I will fear no evil: for thou art with me; thy rod and thy staff they comfort me. Thou preparest a table before me in the presence of mine enemies: thou anointest my head with oil; my cup runneth over" (Psalm 23:4-5, KJV). It is only when God allows us to experience some hardship and difficulty that we can comprehend the meaning of the words from Andraé Crouch, who once observed, "If I never had a problem, I would not know that God could solve them."[2]

It may sound strange for me to say this, but I now thank God for what I have been through this past year. Why? Because now, like Paul, I am persuaded that God is in the blessing business.

I am persuaded that God is in the healing business.

I am persuaded that God is in the prayer-hearing and the prayer-answering business.

I am persuaded that God can guide the hands of surgeons and can take your cancer away.

I am persuaded that weeping can endure for an evening but joy comes in the morning.

I am persuaded that earth has no sorrow that heaven cannot heal.

I am persuaded!

All of my life, I have heard other people say these things in prayer meeting, but until last year, I had not had an IV hooked up to my arm and a catheter extending from my body while I was confined to a hospital bed. I didn't have the scar of an incision that greeted me every morning when I looked in the mirror. I didn't have a disease spreading through my body that had the ability to end my life at the age of fifty-four. Prior to 2003, I was just listening to what God had been doing in the lives of others.

Today I am in a different spiritual position. Today I declare to you that I am persuaded. The cancer did not touch any of my lymph nodes or any other organs. I am persuaded. I did not need to have any chemotherapy or radiation therapy. I am persuaded. After six months of knowing that I had cancer, and after six weeks of recovering from surgery to remove the cancer, and after six months of follow-up visits to my surgeon, I am now cancer free. I am persuaded that nothing can, nothing did, and nothing ever will separate me from the love of God. I know for myself, in ways I could never have known before, what the songwriter was feeling when he wrote these words: "He promised never to leave me, Never to leave me alone."[3]

Let me pause here and acknowledge that I fully understand that not everybody will be fortunate enough to have my experience of being healed from cancer. For some people, their cancer is still attacking them. Their problems have not been resolved. Their pillow may still be stained from the tears they shed last night. If you are one of these people, I want to remind you that just because your trials have not yet ended, it does not mean that God is not present. Keep your hand in God's hand and let God bring you through whatever storm may be raging in your life.

You are not passing through it by yourself. God is able to sustain you, uphold you, and even carry you for as long as you need divine strength upon which to lean. Believe the Scriptures when they say that nothing can separate you from the love of God. Believe Jesus when he promises never to fail or forsake you. And believe me when I tell you that I am persuaded like never before that God will keep his promise and he will never leave you alone.

NOTES

1. Jennie Wilson, "Hold to God's Unchanging Hand," *African American Heritage Hymnal* (Chicago: GIA, 2001), p. 404.
2. Andraé Crouch, "Through It All," *The Best of Lift Him Up*, Benson Music Group: Nashville, TN, 1994, p. 133.
3. Nolan Williams Jr., "Never Alone," *African American Heritage Hymnal* (Chicago: GIA, 2001), p. 310.

Bibliography

American Cancer Society. *Cancer Facts and Figures, 2003*.
———. *Facts on Prostate and Prostate Cancer Testing, 2002*.
———. *Guidelines for the Early Detection of Prostate Cancer, 2002*.

Chappell, Kevin. "Dr. Ben Carson: Top Surgeon's Life-and-Death Struggle with Prostate Cancer." *Ebony*, January 2003, pp. 38–42.

———. "Life after Prostate Cancer: NMA and Top Leaders Launch Campaign against Leading Killer of Black Men." *Ebony*, September 2003, pp. 188–90.

Compton, Josette. "African American Men Most Susceptible to Prostate Cancer." *The Call and Post*, January 16, 2004, p. A4.

Heard, Eric. "Practicing What You Preach, Even When It Is Done from the Valley of the Shadow of Death." *The Call and Post*, magazine supplement, August 7, 2003, pp. 8–9.

Klein, Eric A., ed. *Management of Prostate Cancer*, 2nd ed. Totowa, NJ: Humana, 2004.

Kushner, Harold. *When Bad Things Happen to Good People*. New York: Avon, 1981.

Marks, Sheldon. *Prostate and Cancer: A Family Guide to Diagnosis, Treatment, and Survival*. Cambridge, MA: Fisher, 1995.

McFarland, John Robert. *Now That I Have Cancer—I Am Whole: Meditations for Cancer Patients and Those Who Love Them*. Kansas City, MO: Andrews & McMeel, 1993.

Oesterling, Joseph E., and Mark A. Moyad. *The ABCs of Prostate Cancer: The Book That Could Save Your Life*. Lanham, MD: Madison, 1997.

Phillips, Robert H. *Coping with Prostate Cancer: A Guide to Living with Prostate Cancer for You and Your Family*. Garden City, NY: Avery, 1994.

Parker-Pope, Tara. "To Improve Prostate Cancer Detection, Doctors Change Approach to Testing." *The Wall Street Journal*, March 23, 2004, Health Journal Section, p. 10.

Sanders, Buffy. *The Prostate Diet Cookbook: Cancer-Fighting Foods for a Healthy Prostate*. Gig Harbor, WA: Harbor, 2001.

Seard, Leon. "What's a Man to Do?" *Message*, March–April 2003, p. 22–27.

Shames, Laurence, and Peter Barton. *Not Fade Away: A Short Life Well Lived*. New York: Rodale, 2003.

Strum, Stephen B., and Donna L. Pogliano. *A Primer on Prostate Cancer: The Empowered Patient's Guide*. Hollywood, FL: Life Extension Media, 2002.

Tanner, Lindsey. "Study Suggests Radiation as Prostate Cancer Cure." *The Plain Dealer*, March 17, 2004, p.A11.

Teplinsky, Michael. *Complete Guide to Prostate Health*. Physicians' Choice, 2002. 1-888-287-3800.

Thomas, Frank A. *The Lord's Prayer: In Times Such as These*. St. Louis: Chalice, 2002.

Vergano, Dan. "Improved PSA Test Means Fewer False Positives, Less Controversy." *USA Today*, October 23, 2003, p. D1.

Walsh, Patrick, and Janet Farrar Worthington. *Dr. Patrick Walsh's Guide to Surviving Prostate Cancer*. New York: Warner, 2001.

———. *The Prostate: A Guide for Men and the Women Who Love Them*. New York: Warner, 1997.

Notes

If you are battling prostate cancer, please consider using the following pages to record your thoughts, feelings, and plans.

♦♦ What feelings and thoughts have been most prominent in my mind?

♦♦ What steps have I taken so far?

◆◆ What additional steps might I take?

◆◆ What support systems are available to me?

◆◆ How can I take advantage of these support systems?

Notes

❧ What questions do I still have about this disease?

❧ How can I get these questions answered?

❧ How has my faith made a difference in this struggle?

❧ How might I use my experience to help other men (and their families) who are battling prostate cancer?

❧ Additional Thoughts